EMOTIONAL SELF-CARE FOR BLACK WOMEN

DISCOVER HOW TO RAISE YOUR SELF-ESTEEM,
ELIMINATE NEGATIVE THINKING AND HEAL FROM
PAST TRAUMAS EVEN IF YOUR LIFE IS CHAOTIC
RIGHT NOW

ALICIA MAGORO

CONTENTS

INTRODUCTION

Do not judge me by my success, judge me by how many times I fell down and got back up again.

— NELSON MANDELA

WHAT SOCIETY WANTS, SOCIETY GETS

As a woman, society expects so much from you. Not only should you be accomplished as a family woman, but some will also expect you to be educated as well. As much as we may be considered the weaker sex, we are anything but. A woman in the 21st century is expected to do a lot more than to birth and raise her children. No, it is not enough to stand before a stove and prepare hot meals for your family every single night, you need to also be an amazing and attentive lover.

A woman must also look impeccable as she juggles seven roles. She should never forget that she is the nurturer, who cooks and cares for the home and her family. The house must be neat at all times, no matter how many children live in it. But to be a powerful woman, she is also expected to earn her place in the corporate world and be a financial contributor in her home. All bills must be paid; if she falls short, she has to make a plan. There are so many requirements, and you can end up feeling stretched thin because you serve as a lover, a cleaner, a maid, a cook, a nurse, a therapist, or whatever else your family needs you to be at that moment. It is a lot.

Being overwhelmed is a state of being most women are used to existing in. If you vent to another woman, they may sympathize, but they will probably tell you ways to cope with your load without telling you how to care for yourself. Women prioritize their parents, their children, their partners, and sometimes even their jobs, before themselves. We don't know how to put ourselves first, and if we do manage to do so, we feel guilty that we made a decision based solely on what we want. So much depends on us and what we do; therefore, we feel terrified to take time for ourselves, because what will be the fate of all the people and things that depend on us?

WE DON'T KNOW SELF-CARE

Black women do not take the time to care for themselves emotionally. They do not step away from their busy schedules to replenish their emotional reserves that are running on empty. Frankly, we do not know how to step away or take a break. We keep going and do whatever it takes to keep sane, healthy, and relatively content and happy. Unfortunately, that is not enough. What is at risk of deteriorating is our mental health. When your mental health is in shambles, you are running the risk of affecting the state of your physical health and spirituality.

In life, all the elements are connected: The air is connected to the water and the land. They all rely on and affect the other. This is true about your body. Your spirituality is connected to your mental state, which is also connected to your physical being. They are all in sync with one another such that if one of them is off, it will wreak havoc on the others. Take note of all the times you had troubles with your spirituality or mental health; somehow it manifested physically. The same care we give our bodies by exercising and eating right, we need to afford our emotional, spiritual, and mental health. Our health is holistic and includes our minds and emotional health.

I think because we keep going, we think we are okay. Our lives and the stability within them depend on our emotions and how we are handling them. We will not have the patience or vigor to take care of the home or the children when our emotional strength is spent. Have you ever noticed how irritable you become when you are at your wit's end emotionally? The smallest inconvenience feels like a mountain to get over and things that do not usually bother you make you want to tear your hair out in frustration. Emotions play a significant role and dictate how much frustration you can take on a daily basis and your resilience during these times.

WE ARE NOT TAUGHT COPING SKILLS

Black mothers and grandmothers all around the world lived in a time where they could not go to school and better themselves. They were taught to rely on men for their well-being and, in turn, they had to smile and bear the brunt of abusive treatment. Whether it was abuse from their fathers, uncles, brothers, or husbands, black women were at the mercy of men. There was no way out, so they learnt to survive and suck it up. The generations that existed in the height of female oppression knew they had to be seen and not heard and do what they needed to cope. Crying or giving up was seen as a weakness; they believed the weak would perish. These women that raised us were tough as nails and they could weather any storm.

We were raised on survival. Emotions were a waste of time because as a woman, you still had a role to play. Having never seen the maternal figures in our lives break down, we were taught never to show emotion, and that letting your emotions get the better of you was a weakness. We are never really taught how to confront how we feel and we grow up smothering our emotions and only letting them escape as anger or other self-preservation techniques, like always having your guard up and not trusting anyone.

Due to our inability to properly deal with our emotions because we were never taught how to, there is a bias and stigma around black women and our emotions. The angry black woman is a common one. We are also labeled as sassy or full of attitude. Society can portray us as emotionally unhinged, and people will believe it. It is sad, because we are more than this one-dimensional portrayal. Our emotional outbursts may occur more often because we have so much on our plates.

The black single mother is expected to provide and nurture without feeling the emotional strain. The black employee should work happily without feeling discriminated against, although there are clear biases against her. A black woman has little support and no healthy outlets to release her frustrations. It is an uphill battle for us to be given the respect due to us or the credit we deserve for all our accomplishments. It is difficult not to be frustrated when all we do is make winning moves and yet we never win.

BREAK FREE

The stigma that currently surrounds us does not have to hold us down. As black women, we can show the world that we are more than what we are perceived as. Sometimes we are weighed down by the stigma that is attached to our beautiful black skin; it can get heavy when it feels like the world does not care about you. Fortunately, you have the opportunity every day to choose to break free of the stigma. You have self-control and can decide to react differently to stressful situations. You can be a fighter and show love at the same time. But this can only be achieved when we are able to face and master our emotions.

When we fail to control our emotions, they are in control. They will dictate your reactions and how you respond to the way life is unfolding around you. When you are experiencing a lot of positive emotions then it is not so bad; the problem becomes when you are being controlled by negative emotions like fear, mistrust, and anger. Leading with those kinds of emotions will erode your quality of life in a way that can end up breaking you. You don't want to be controlled by resentment, guilt, shame, or frustration. Your actions will be fueled by anger because you will tire quite quickly.

When negative emotions are in the driver's seat of your life, it will bring you down. You will have a negative mindset, which will also bring down your willpower to overcome obstacles and carry on in life. Having a deeper under-standing of your emotions means that you know how to accurately respond to situations and how to act in an appro-priate manner. After processing how you feel, you will also know how to recover and make yourself feel better in spite of the circumstances. Suppressing emotions and neglecting our emotional welfare only leads to disaster.

YOUR FEELINGS ARE POWER

Feeling what you feel with your entire being is not a weak-ness, it is a power. When we are happy, we do not run from those feelings; we fully immerse ourselves in feelings of happiness, we do not even question or suppress them. When you start feeling an unpleasant emotion, lean into it. This is how you unlock the power within you. As an authentic being, there will be good and bad within you coexisting peacefully; you will also feel good and bad things, it is a part of the human experience. Allowing yourself to feel every-thing lets you know when you are not coping and may need help and support.

When you suppress your negative emotions, you are not able to gauge what you can and cannot handle. Think of it as lifting weights. You know you can lift a 45 lbs. dumbbell because you have tried and succeeded at doing so. You know you can't lift a 90 lbs. dumbbell because you have tried and failed at doing so; you know you will need help lifting it. When it comes to handling your emotions, how will you know what you can handle if you do not ever try to handle your emotions? How will you know what your limit is and when you will need to ask for help?

Your feelings are not annoying. If you allow them into your life, they will show you things that you may have been oblivious to. When you are suffering a physical ailment, it manifests as a symptom, and that is true of your emotional health as well. The way you feel is a vital indication of your mental and emotional well-being. The emotional sensations that you are running from or suppressing are what will essentially tell you whether or not you are okay.

YOUR EMOTIONS ARE TOOLS

If you change your mindset, your emotions will no longer be scary to you. Rather, you will view them as tools you can use to motivate you to keep going. If you think you will not be able to achieve this paradigm shift, do not worry, this is where this book will help you. You will learn to use your emotions as tools to energize and revitalize your purpose in life. Moreover, you can weaponize your emotions and use them as fuel to go for what you want. For example, a lot of people who lose weight do not only do it for their health, but they also use how they felt when they were ridiculed for being overweight as a motivating tool to reach their goal weight.

As a black woman, if you were told you were too confrontational or too angry or too loud, use how you felt when you were being put down as fuel to do better. Use those emotions to lift yourself higher and gain a deeper understanding of yourself. You have everything you need in order to unlock a higher understanding of how you function as an emotional being. After achieving this understanding, you will achieve a better quality of life and begin to act in a way that is more enlightened. Sharpen your tools so you can use them to achieve emotional strength.

Perhaps you once knew how to use your emotions in order to improve your life but have since lost touch with those skills. When you don't use the tools that are available to you, they can become dull over time or rusted. Neglecting your emotions means you will not be able to adequately interpret the messages they bring. You won't know why you are angered by certain things or why you get frustrated in other situations. When your tools are not in the best condition, it is difficult to use them. You will be doomed to misunderstand your own emotions and base your decisions on an erroneous thought process.

WHAT WILL THIS BOOK DO?

You are reading this book because you may not have the right tools to face your emotions and manage them in a healthy way. You may have run from how you felt and made every excuse not to face what you feel. You might procrastinate on giving yourself the emotional self-care that you deserve. That behavior ends today. You no longer have to live in fear or jump through hoops pretending your emotions do not phase you. We know you care, and I do too. I want to reveal to you what you can do in order to handle your emotions and come out better as a black woman.

As you page through this book, it will give you the basic foundation of what it means to master emotional self-care. A powerful woman is one who has mastered herself, and that is what this book aims to achieve. I want to give you everything you will need in order to gain an understanding of what your emotions are and how you can manage them so that you can breeze through the obstacles that are present in everyday life. Included within these pages are practical ways to implement self-care in such a way that it is woven into your daily habits.

Your destiny does not rely on a life that is restricted by bias, discrimination, and stigma. Black women in history have continuously defied expectations and risen above what society thought of them. Black women have shown their resilience and power century after century. You do not have to fear not being good enough because you have always been enough. Your fate is greater than your emotional shortcomings. You are bigger than your weaknesses and stronger than the discrimination you experience.

Emotional self-care is a commitment that you need to make to yourself every day. Just because it is something good for you does not mean it won't be hard work. You have to pour yourself into this self-improvement phase so that whatever self-improvement methods and techniques you implement in your life will work. You are on the precipice of change. It may feel terrifying, exhilarating, and emotional. You'll be feeling things you've been avoiding for a long time. It may get dark before you see any kind of light at the end of the tunnel. Trust the process and you will get there.

Imagine not feeling burdened by the expectations of the society and not really caring what anyone thinks about you. Imagine knowing your true self and understanding how to manage your emotions. Wouldn't that be liberating? It is time for you to take control of your emotional health and begin feeling powerful from within. The time is now to shed your emotional baggage and equip yourself with the power inherent in your emotions. Do not leave it for tomorrow; today begins your journey of self-care and developing powerful emotional strengths.

1

EMOTIONS AS HELPFUL MESSENGERS

Follow your feelings. If it feels right, move forward. If it doesn't feel right, don't do it.

— OPRAH WINFREY

HOW YOUR BODY CREATES THE FEELING OF EMOTION

According to the APA Dictionary of Psychology (n.d.), emotion is defined as "a complex reaction pattern, involving experiential, behavioral, and physiological elements, by which an individual attempts to deal with a personally significant matter or event." The specific details of the event will determine your emotion; if the event is one where you receive disapproval from a loved one, you may experience shame, whereas if the event is one where your safety is put under threat, then you are likely to feel fear. But how do you generate these feelings?

Your emotions are sensations that you experience with your body. These sensations begin on a biological level. A lot of strides have been made in neuroscience and it can be concluded that the sensations that create emotions emanate from the brain. Unlike what was theorized in past misconceptions, we now know emotions are not located in certain parts of the brain. We now know that the same emotion can be achieved via different networks in the brain. Although different networks in the brain can lead to the same emotion, your brain has created certain sensations for each emotion.

When you experience something, your brain will allocate various sensations to what you are going through. If you are ever in a similar scenario, you may experience the same sensations and emotions. There are core networks in the brain that will essentially contribute to various feelings (sadness, happiness, surprise, anger) at various levels. Essentially, the sensations emanate from various chemical reactions within the brain as well as hormones; the sensations flood your system and create bodily reactions, like the lump in your throat when you are upset or that fluttering feeling in your belly when you are anxious about something. In short, thoughts can create certain chemical reactions, which in turn create feelings.

YOU ARE NOT WHAT YOU FEEL

Each person experiences life differently from the next person. There may be feelings you experience more often than the next person. Perhaps, due to the circumstances in your life, you experience anger more than the average person; are you now an angry person? Maybe the emotion you identify with is happy; does that make you a happy person? The good news is that you are not what you feel; your feelings serve as an extension of your human experience. Sometimes we have a hard time dealing with our feelings because we think that they reveal who we are.

Feelings are how you react to external stimuli. Due to the fact that your feelings are essentially reactions, you may not always have control over how you feel. The only thing you may have control over are your actions. When you experience a certain emotion, you should do your best to separate your identity as a person from what you are feeling. It would not be healthy to attach yourself to certain emotions, especially if they are negative. Imagine how depressed you would become if you attached your identity to your feelings of disappointment, sadness, and discontentment.

The emotions you feel in certain situations do not define who you are as a person because your identity is a permanent aspect and emotions are fleeting. How you feel in the morning is likely to be different to how you feel in the evening because various things happen throughout the day that influence your emotions. You may wake up happy and ready to conquer the day, but then quickly become discouraged by a toxic boss who puts your ideas down. If you tie your identity to how you feel, it may affect you negatively on a day-to-day basis. Feelings that could be easily dealt with will then become exaggerated and intensely felt. There is no need to make mountains out of mole hills.

Feelings do not last. Depending on the situation, feelings can last from an hour to a few days. Nothing you feel is permanent and can be dealt with. Being mindful about your life can help ground you in the present and save you from dwelling on past feelings or emotions. It is important to separate yourself from your feelings and deal with emotions as they arise by dissecting the cause or the thoughts that created those feelings. When you understand where those feelings emanated from, you are more likely to accept those feelings and make a commitment to move forward in a healthy way.

EMOTIONS ARE INDICATORS

Living in a mindful state allows you to be in tune with the changes in your emotions. Being aware of how you feel and how those feelings are affected by certain scenarios or changes in the environment allows you to get a better indication of who you are. Based on your thoughts, you may have a perception of who you think you are, but that is not necessarily who you are. "My thoughts are my own but they do not describe me. Because I think or feel anxious, that doesn't mean that I am anxious. It means I am experiencing the symptoms of anxiety, not that I am anxiety" (Parry, 2014).

When you have the ability to notice the change, then you have the power to control how you react. When you're not self-aware of your emotions and your behavior, you are not in control of your reactions. If you consistently allow yourself to experience all your emotions then it gives you more choice over how to react, because you have noticed everything that you are feeling and have accepted those emotions. Denial and suppression create room for unpredictable reactions. When you notice your feelings and how they evolve and change, it also gives you the power to pause before acting.

As a black woman, you go through an array of emotions on a daily basis. If your body is experiencing a medical crisis, your body will show you that something is wrong by manifesting physical symptoms. When the symptoms show up, you know that there is something you need to sort out. Your emotions serve the same function as your symptoms because they are indicators of your emotional state. When you feel your emotions changing do not run, but rather take note, and you will learn something about yourself.

Be intrigued by your emotions, because studying them can reveal a lot about your inner health. Think of yourself as a scientist and become educated in yourself and what your emotions mean. When these uncomfortable feelings arise, ask yourself the following:

1. Is there anything that I can provide my physical being to make it feel better? Will rest/food/warmth/care help ease what I am feeling now?
2. What thoughts were running through my mind that may have contributed to this emotion?

SEPARATE AWARENESS

Divorcing your identity from your thoughts and emotions is a powerful experience that will kickstart your spiritual awakening. Your thoughts seemingly arise out of nowhere and present themselves to your mind as they are. If you take a step back and immerse yourself in meditation, you will notice that they do this randomly and you have no idea what will arise next. The thoughts and emotions come to the fore of your mind, linger, then move aside for the next thoughts.

When you allow your mind to be empty, you will soon realize that your mind has a "mind of its own," because it often wanders and creates its own thoughts. If you removed your thoughts, what would be left in your consciousness? When you strip yourself of your memories, ideas, and beliefs, what is left? This 'you' that exists after all forms of thought are stripped from it is what is called "separate awareness," and some think of it as your soul or true being. To ask who is there when your thoughts are not present will lead you to the question of who the observer is when you let go.

If you take time to meditate and live in the now, you will have the opportunity to empty yourself of all the knowledge you have about what exists in the world. This means that when you remove from your conscience all memories of good and bad, you will learn who is there in the moment. After putting aside all thought, who remains? When you exist only in the present you will get to know a version of yourself that is stripped of pride or shame and that is devoid of any self-judgment. As you meditate, what 'you' is left?

After taking a step back, who is the one observing? It is interesting to observe yourself as you take a step back. You can see how you are, how thoughts arise and how they pass, what feelings arise and which ones linger. This observation of self allows you to separate yourself and see how you exist in the now. It can also be liberating to exist without thought and the burden of your ideas and perceptions. Without the mask of expectations and past knowledge and experience, you will experience the true essence of yourself. Do you feel empty as you detach from your thoughts? Do you feel light, peaceful, aware?

You may experience difficulty trying to divorce yourself from your thoughts. If you perform an experiment, you may be able to let go of thoughts more easily. The Sedona method demonstrates how easy it is to let go of your feelings and thoughts because they do not form a part of you. Hale Dwoskin gives a powerful analogy of the relationship you have with your mind. Roll a pen back and forth in your palm; the pen is any feelings, thoughts, or emotions you may be feeling in the moment and represents you and your awareness in the moment.

You should be aware that, though the pen is in your hand, it is not a part of you, nor is it attached to you in any way. The pen is like your feelings, thoughts, or emotions that temporarily arise in your awareness. Close your fingers around the pen and grip it; this is what happens when you attach your identity to thoughts and struggle against them. Now turn your fist to face the floor and release your grip on the pen so that it falls to the ground. The pen was only in your hand and never a part of it, so you can release it at any time. Your thoughts, feelings, and emotions may be a part of your awareness in the moment, but they are not who you are, even when you identify with them.

If your thoughts and feelings were a part of you, you would not be able to let them go, they would be present all the time. Happiness, sadness, anger, and any other emotion comes and goes as we go through life. Instead of experiencing these feelings when they arise and letting go of them when they leave, we hang on to them and attach our identities to them. If someone does something that hurts us, instead of saying, "I am feeling hurt and angry," we say, "I am hurt; I am angry". "You suffer, not because anger or sadness is present, but because you mistake temporary states as being who you are. You personalize them and suffer as a result" (Paterson, 2022).

LET'S MEDITATE

Perhaps you have not been able to separate yourself from your thoughts because you have not taken the time to meditate and find the answers. Meditation can seem terrifying if you are used to trying to escape yourself and how you feel. In order to truly understand yourself and how you feel, meditation will become a part of the process. Mindful meditation "involves the state of being aware of and involved in the present moment and making yourself open, aware, and accepting" (Cherry, 2020). I want you to be able to observe your thoughts and feelings. Observing your feelings means you are existing within them and not trying to ignore or deny them.

After observing your feelings, the next step is to track them by writing them down. Once you have written them down, over a period of time, you may be able to spot patterns and discern where negative feelings are coming from. When you are able to track the genesis of bad thoughts and feelings, you will be able to solve a lot of your problems or be assertive about certain situations. When you feel bad after every time you think about your job, perhaps you are in a toxic work environment and you need to start thinking about removing yourself from it. This guided mindful meditation will help you to observe your thoughts; do this on a daily basis then write down what you felt when certain thoughts come to mind.

Mindful Meditation

1. Find a comfortable place to sit or lay down; it doesn't matter if you are sitting or lying down, as long as you will not be disturbed and you are comfortable.
2. Take a deep breath in and hold it for a few seconds; exhale with the intent of letting go of all thought. Repeat this ten times.
3. As you continue your deep breathing, think of yourself in the now as you are today, without a past or a future or gender or social status. Think of yourself as a soul essence.
4. Empty yourself of your earthly presence and observe what remains. Who are you when the concepts of thought and identity have been removed?
5. Allow your mind to wander and observe the thoughts that spontaneously occur; how do they make you feel?

Thoughts That Do Not Help

Sometimes you can get stuck in a thought loop pattern that is negative or that makes you dread facing your thoughts. Identifying your thought patterns can reveal why you keep getting stuck in the same emotions. Preconceived ideas may lead to negative emotions, but perhaps that is not even what is happening; because you are stuck in the thought pattern, your experiences will always be the same. You may have a 'My mother does not approve of me' pattern, or a 'My boss does not believe in me' pattern, or a 'Men can never be trusted' thought pattern.

In order to have better experiences that are not directly influenced by these thought patterns, you have to recognize that they are there. When you have done that, you will have more control when you see your mind going into that thought pattern. You will not immediately act on them and can separate yourself from them to assess if what you think is really happening or if it is in your mind. Let go of these patterns and introduce ideas and opinions that are opposite to these thought patterns. Instead of thinking, 'My mother does not approve of me', think rather, 'My mother only wants the best for me.' When you introduce new ideas, you will also recognize when your thought patterns are leading you to negative emotions.

DO NOT BE AFRAID

At the end of the day, your feelings are not going anywhere. It is counterproductive to run from them or try to suppress them. Learning to identify your feelings is a strength that will add value to your life. Your feelings are tools you can use to make better decisions in your life. When you are in the dark, your feelings can be the lighthouse that guides you to enlightenment. There is nothing to fear. Even if your feelings are not pleasant, they are fleeting, temporary, and will not last forever. Think of your feelings as uncomfortable shoes; at some point, you will get to take them off. If you are struggling to face what you feel, read on—the tools you need to understand what you feel and why are just ahead.

2

GETTING TO KNOW YOUR FEELINGS

Your intellect may be confused, but your emotions will never lie to you.

— ROGER EBERT

In the previous chapter, we established that emotions are helpful messengers that bring you helpful information that you can use to make more informed decisions about your life. Moreover, your emotions give you the opportunity to know yourself better. As a black woman, you often carry the weight of the world on your shoulders. You have to try to keep your femininity and stay attractive and put together. At the same time, you have to be bold and daring while going after your career goals. As a mother and lover, you have to keep your nurturing side so that you can keep your home a warm and loving place. You have to do so much for everyone else, but you should not forget to put yourself first.

Putting yourself as a priority in your life is easier said than done. We often ignore our own feelings for the greater good. We ignore our own feelings of unhappiness, dissatisfaction, and disappointment, often to keep the peace at home. We suppress feelings of rage at work when we are overlooked for promotion. We switch off the messages our feelings are sending us so that we do not have to stand up for ourselves. This is just one scenario. It can happen that you absolutely do not know the messages your emotions are sending you. You might not understand why you are jealous, angry, or upset. Why would you feel that way?

In order to receive the messaging inherent in your feelings and emotions, you need to be able to identify what emotions you are feeling. Not every woman is aware of every emotion, and not everyone is adept at identifying when they are feeling which emotion. To identify your emotions is important so that you are able to further understand why you feel the way you do. This chapter will be dedicated to getting to understand your feelings and to identify the root emotion. By the end of the chapter, you will be able to name your feelings and to understand what primary and secondary emotions are. We will also get into the topic of uncomfortable emotions and how to experience them without running.

Getting to know your emotions is a way to empower yourself because once you are able to identify your emotions, there is so much you can learn. A black woman is forever evolving and becoming the best that she can be. This kind of knowledge allows you to unlock parts of yourself that you didn't even know existed. Have you ever been surprised at your own strength and capabilities? Have you ever doubted yourself but came out victorious in the end? This is not solely based on luck; unexpected success is often because we doubt ourselves. How we feel about ourselves may be wrong because we misinterpret our emotions.

HOW TO UNDERSTAND THE MESSAGE BEHIND THE EMOTION

To decipher the messages that your emotions are attempting to communicate with you, you have to first ask yourself what emotion you are feeling. Only after correctly identifying the emotion you are feeling can you put it into context and interpret it correctly. You may not have the necessary tools to identify the root emotion and therefore, you may need to practice the skill a few times. There are certain things that you can do and practice in order to get better at identifying your emotions.

Acknowledging and Labeling Your Feelings

Life doesn't come at you slowly, giving you time to process. Sometimes things come at you quickly and it is difficult to decipher what you are feeling. Your bad day could become a bad week, and that bad week could become a bad month. Sometimes you feel a mixture of things that are good and bad. At the end of the day, you should be able to notice how your feelings and emotions shift and define what you are feeling at a particular time. Acknowledging how you feel is noticing how your feelings may change from one moment to the next.

Your feelings change depending on so many different things. You may feel refreshed and energized when coming back from a vacation. You may feel annoyed because you were stuck in gridlock traffic on your way to work. You might feel relaxed as you stream your favorite television show with your dog at your feet. These feelings will change based on what you're doing and who you're doing it with; acknowledge how you feel as your life unfolds before you. Sometimes it's not very easy to acknowledge how you feel because you don't know what you are feeling.

The best thing to help you identify your feelings is a feelings chart. Children are usually given feelings charts in order to educate them about their emotions, and so that they can recognize certain bodily sensations and communicate them adequately. Children are taught this so that they can be further taught how to deal with their emotions via healthy coping mechanisms. As an adult, you may also benefit from using a feelings chart in order to notice and name your feelings. If you have never come across a feelings chart, you may be a little lost as to what I am referring to.

A feelings chart displays various feelings that you may experience; the feelings on the chart can include happy, sad, angry, scared, shy, confident, surprised, ashamed, disgusted, exhausted, confused, bored, and so on. If you are making the feelings chart yourself, then there is no limit to the emotions that you can include on it. You can print one from the internet or you can make one yourself on some cardboard with some colored markers. You can really have fun with it if you like. When you have completed it, it can be used to aid you in identifying how you feel at certain moments.

Practice With One Emotion at a Time

Life is filled with so many complicated emotions. In order not to get overwhelmed by your emotions, it's better to take things slow and work on one emotion at a time. You could do this on a daily or weekly basis. Choose one emotion, such as gratefulness. Track this emotion for the amount of time that suits you. Notice when you begin to feel grateful; what is the gratitude directed at? Picture the word in your mind and repeat it to yourself. Write down every time you feel grateful. To what degree did you feel grateful? Was it an intense feeling or was it a mild one?

Once you have sufficiently tracked an emotion, reflect on it and what it meant to you. Was it a good emotion for you or was it a bad emotion? Do you want to feel the emotion again? You can mind map everything you think about the emotions; write the emotion and draw a circle around it, then draw branches that you will use to write a description of what that emotion means to you. Do not be afraid to delve deeper into the emotion. Once you have thoroughly explored the emotion, you can move onto the next one.

Use Synonyms

There are so many different words to say 'happy.' Try to attach various words to the same emotion and see how many you can name. Synonyms for the word happy include joyful, cheery, delighted, gleeful, jovial, content, and merry. There are so many different ways to say that you are happy because there are different levels to happiness. Emotion is like a spectrum; therefore, you can feel it at varying degrees, and you can express it as such. Being happy that your dog did not urinate on the carpet is not the same as being happy that you have graduated from college.

Using synonyms is helpful in getting to know your emotions because it allows you to give the emotion color. You can get so angry that you yell at someone; saying you yelled in anger will express that you were angry and you yelled, but saying you yelled in exasperation shows that you were so angry, you yelled because you were at the end of your tether. Synonyms allow you to be more descriptive with how you feel, and this is helpful because emotions can be complicated and vast.

Journal About Your Feelings

A journal allows you to keep a record of where you began and where you are now. This is beneficial when you are trying to get to know your emotions. When you put a pen to paper, or make any other record of how you feel, you stop to think about what you are writing down; when you're heated up, your emotions just drive your hands and mind to pour out what you really feel. Keeping a journal about your feelings can give you insights about emotional patterns and what your triggers are. It is important for your emotional development to journal about your feelings.

Pick a time that is suitable to you, either in the morning or in the evening, when you can sit undisturbed and jot down how you are feeling. Not only should you journal about your feelings, but you can also explore the cause of those feelings and map how you arrived there. Journaling is not necessarily just writing down how you feel; you can choose to make music, paint, write poetry, or any other artistic medium that helps you express your feelings. Words can be difficult to articulate, so use whatever method you feel most comfortable with to express your emotions regularly.

Feelings Are All Around You

Art imitates life. Feelings are not only seen in people around you, such as your family and colleagues, but they can also be witnessed in art such as songs, movies, and books. When you are watching a movie, take note of how they show emotion.

The actors will not scream about how frustrated they are, but rather show it through the art of acting. They may punch a wall, break a glass, or tear a newspaper into pieces and then storm off into the darkness. You may notice it via subtle cues like clenching of that fist at their side, or their jaw.

Getting to know your feelings means observing how song-writers use melodic tones and lyrics to express love, happiness, or heartbreak. Can you feel what they feel? Does it bring back similar emotions? Listening to music or watching movies that depict scenes that are similar to what you have gone through can be quite an intense experience, as it can force you to relive those memories that made you experience the emotions being expressed. This is a part of getting to know your emotions.

PRIMARY AND SECONDARY EMOTIONS

Emotions are experienced by every person in every culture. Primary emotions are the first and direct reactions you feel in a situation. They are said to be primary emotions as they are what comes first. When something occurs, your very first reaction alerts you to what your needs may be in that scenario. For example, if your loved one is threatened, your immediate emotional reaction is to get angry, and then you may feel the need to protect them and set boundaries. In that situation, anger is your primary emotion.

If your loved one has been threatened by somebody that you care about, this may create feelings of sadness. With the secondary emotion, sadness has resulted from you reacting to the primary emotion of anger. You are sad because you have to get angry at someone who threatened someone else you love. Imagine if your spouse threatened your parents; you would definitely feel angry and then sad. Sometimes secondary emotions are misleading and cover up what you actually feel.

Primary Emotions

The boom of psychology as a science in the 1970s saw many psychologists make advancements in terms of theories about feelings. One such psychologist was Paul Eckman, who identified six primary emotions that are experienced by every person. The emotions Eckman identified were sadness, happiness, fear, disgust, anger, and surprise. He later added shame, pride, excitement, and embarrassment to this list of basic emotions. Primary emotions can also act as secondary emotions.

It is important to note that emotions can be combined much like colors. Robert Plutschik came up with a wheel of emotions that functions similar to how a color wheel works: If you mix two emotions, they can create another. Based on this theory the basic emotions may be used much like building blocks to lead to more complex emotions. If you combine two basic emotions such as trust and joy, you can create love. Instead of thinking of emotions as distinct from one another, it is perhaps better to understand emotions as a gradient. A person can experience one singular emotion or a mixture of two or more.

Secondary Emotions

Primary emotions can also act as secondary emotions, and some secondary emotions are more prevalent than others. The more typical secondary emotions include irritation, anxiety, global depressed mood, aggression, emptiness or hopelessness, and rage. Secondary emotions are what you feel about the primary emotion itself; these types of feelings can be hard to understand and interpret. They linger and last for much longer than primary emotions and include feelings of shame, guilt, frustration, remorse, and resentment.

Secondary emotions are more complex and therefore will increase the intensity of how you feel the primary emotions. Your secondary emotion can lead to you feeling discomfort with your primary emotion, an identity crisis, a trauma trigger, or emotions tied to your fears about the future. In order to be able to cope sufficiently in life, you need to be able to discern between a primary emotion and a secondary one.

How to Differentiate Between Primary and Secondary Emotions

There are various questions you may ask yourself in order to decipher whether your emotion is a primary or a secondary one:

1. Ask yourself if the emotion is tied to external stimuli that you observed or that happened to you. If the answer is yes, the emotion is primary.
2. Ask yourself if you are feeling the emotion more intensely as time passes. If the answer is yes, then it is a secondary emotion.
3. Ask yourself if you experience the emotion more times than the event that evoked the emotion. If the answer is yes, then the emotion is a secondary one.
4. Ask yourself if the emotion went away when the event that caused it stopped. If the answer is yes, the emotion is a primary.
5. Ask yourself if the emotion sticks with you beyond the present and affects your abilities as well as hindering your experiences. If the answer is yes, then it is a secondary emotion.
6. Ask yourself if the emotion is complicated, hard to grasp, and ambiguous. If the answer is yes, then it is a secondary emotion.

UNCOMFORTABLE EMOTION

Emotions are a spectrum and therefore, there will be some that we are uncomfortable with. Perhaps you feel guilt or shame because you felt a certain way in a given scenario. It is not always easy to sit with those emotions and accept that you felt that way at that time. Uncomfortable emotions often point toward an unmet need; to understand the message the uncomfortable feeling is sending you; you have to sit in the emotion and attempt to unravel the chaos. Sitting within your feelings, practicing mindfulness, and allowing yourself to truly feel the uncomfortable emotions allows you to flex your emotional muscle, increasing your tolerance of uncomfortable emotions.

Facing your uncomfortable feelings and giving them an opportunity to point to your unmet needs means you are able to practice awareness and use them as valuable data. Human beings have a lot of emotional needs, but the top six include certainty (feeling safe, comfort), significance (feeling unique, special), variety (feeling interest, adventure), love and connection (feeling accepted, supported), contribution (feeling the need to give) and growth (feeling desire to learn, grow).

When any of these emotional needs are not met, or encroached upon, we will have some uncomfortable emotions to deal with. For example, if you want to go to beauty school but your parents would prefer you to study accounting, this means that your need for growth will not be met... You may develop feelings of resentment and frustration. When those feelings arise, it will not help to ignore them. When you slow down and assess where your feelings are pointing you toward, you may increase your chances of getting your emotional needs met.

In light of uncomfortable emotions, you may react in a way that is irrational. When you are reacting irrationally, you may act in that way too. Your energy may not be grounded, and when your energy is in that state, you may not be able to think clearly. Your decision-making will be poor and you may lose the ability to put things into context. To transform your uncomfortable emotions, you need to be aware of what you are feeling first. After identifying what emotions you are feeling, try to understand why you feel the way you do. Once you have understood the why, you can then formulate an action plan of the steps that will help you deal with the issue in a healthy way. In the given example above, you would then create an action plan to show your parents why beauty school is a better fit for you than going to accountancy college. Remember that being vulnerable is power, so it is better to express your emotions rather than to repress them.

THE ROOT OF IT ALL

Getting to the root of your emotions is easier than it sounds. You have to do some considerable digging in order to truly understand where an emotion is rooted. In the beauty school versus accountancy school example, you may think that your frustration is rooted in the fact that your parents always think you are going to fail because you may have let them down before. If you dig further, you will discover the true root of your emotion, which could be that you don't want to be stuck in a dead-end job that is not fulfilling like your parents think it may be.

To get to the root cause of any emotional reaction or feelings, you have to peel back layers where you ask yourself
why over and over until you get to the true root of why you
feel the way you feel. Something that can help in getting to
the root cause of your emotions is keeping a journal. When
you keep account of traumatizing events, you can detail the
specifics of that scenario and why it made you feel the way
you did. You can link this event to other times you felt the
same emotions. Is there a pattern? Can you recall the first
time you experienced this emotion/reaction combination? Is
there a particular trigger?

The reason why you need to understand the root of your
emotions is so that you can stop unhealthy emotional reactions. A lot of emotional reactions are rooted in you feeling a
lack of self-worth. When you are able to identify what the
root cause of your emotional reactions are, you are often
also able to work on neutralizing the trigger. If you are able
to neutralize the trigger, you can unlearn any unhealthy
behavior that you may be using as a coping mechanism.

DIG AND DISCOVER

You have some feelings you have been avoiding because they
may make you uncomfortable. The unpleasant emotions
serve a function too; they are trying to tell you something.
They are screaming at you that something is amiss and that
there is an emotional need of yours that is not being met. If
you ignore your feelings, how will you know what is going

wrong and what needs your attention as soon as possible? You are a powerful woman, who is beginning to be more assertive about her emotions. Take some time and observe how you feel. Why do you feel that way? What could be the cause? Think about any emotionally charged emotions you may have felt recently; do you know what triggered those emotions? Which one of your needs are being stepped on? Is it more than one emotional need that is going unmet? When you have identified what you feel as well as why you feel that way, what will you do with that knowledge? They say knowledge is power; how will you wield your sword?

3

PROCESSING AND RELEASING BIG EMOTIONS

Emotional intelligence is your ability to recognize and understand emotions in yourself and others, and your ability to use this awareness to manage your behavior and relationships.

— TRAVIS BRADBERRY

You are now aware that suppressing your emotions does more harm than good. You have gone through the process of accepting your emotions and being mindful about your everyday life. You have noticed how and when your feelings change and perhaps why they are changing. This is the foundation you need to gain control of your emotions and use them to improve your quality of life. Building upon this foundation, it is important to now learn how to process your emotions.

Your emotions are messages that you have to decipher so that you can understand what they are saying to you. After you get the message, what do you do with it? This chapter is going to equip you with the skills you will need in order to process your emotions, as well as releasing the ones that may be putting you down. Unfortunately, life is not all rainbows and butterflies; life comes with some harsh situations and tough lessons. You have to know when to let go.

PROCESS AND REGULATE

In order to properly receive the messages that our emotions are trying to send us, we should be able as black women to process and regulate our emotions. It is very easy to get carried away in a positive emotion like excitement and do things that end up harming you. The same is true of negative emotions such as anger or resentment; if you are unable to rein in your behavior, you may find that you have acted in a way that is not desirable. Emotional regulation allows us to feel better immediately.

Your long-term well-being is positively affected if you have adequate emotional regulation skills. Feelings of depression or anxiety are less likely to plague you when you can process and regulate your emotions efficiently. There are a host of benefits, such as being able to add value to personal relationships as well as work relationships, and improving your overall health. Emotional regulation is something that most people develop as they grow up. It is a behavioral and mental process that you do, whether consciously or not.

If you did not develop the skill of emotional regulation as you were entering adulthood you can still learn that skill today. In order to cope with life and all the uncertainty it comes with, you should be invested in learning how to regulate your emotions. There are certain practices you can employ in order to regulate your emotions, such as meditation, self-awareness theories, and breathing methods. When you are able to regulate your emotions then those feelings are not likely to escalate into a situation you may regret at a later time.

Your mood is not the same as your emotions, but emotions that are regulated can lead to an improvement in your mood. When you are in a good mood, you are able to be compassionate and empathetic toward others. You are constantly having to face situations and events from the world; not all of them will present themselves positively, therefore, you need to be able to cope and regulate how you feel on a daily basis.

If you are unable to gain control of your emotions and learn how to regulate them, they may create an undesirable situation when you are provoked. If you bottle up unresolved emotions toward someone in your life and fail to deal with them, they can come up in the heat of the moment and you can say or do something that you regret. You may not always be in control and you can easily get overwhelmed by life. There will be times where your emotions spin out of control. It is important that in these moments, you should realize the potential that unmanaged emotion can make your life and those of your loved ones very difficult.

FACE THE STIGMA

Black women are socialized to take on a lot of emotional stress and carry on as if it is not a heavy burden to bear. You are not encouraged to express yourself or complain, but rather to get on with all the things you have to do. This is why the first instinct in us as black women is not necessarily to express ourselves, but rather to suppress and distract ourselves from what we are feeling. We don't want to suppress or avoid our feelings, but our situations don't necessarily allow for expression. If you feel like you have to hold your emotions in, do not do that anymore.

I want to assure you that it is okay to feel things. Any emotion that you feel, whether good or bad, should be felt in its entirety. Do not shut off your feelings. They are a strength. If you suppress your emotions, you are weakening your strength. You may suppress your emotions momentarily, but this act of suppression should not be permanent; at some point you have to address how you feel. If you are suppressing your emotions and not dealing with them at all, that is when it becomes a problem, as you will not be able to regulate yourself adequately.

Why Hide in the First Place?

It is important that we do not approach this issue from a self-righteous pedestal. I offer you my compassion, because you are probably suppressing your feelings for what you deem a good reason. Perhaps this was a way to protect yourself in your past. You may have good intentions around your emotional suppression, but it is not healthy for your emotional state. You may be suppressing your emotions in order to avoid appearing weak. Nobody wants to be judged, and you may feel that if you don't show your true emotions, no one will judge you or use your feelings against you.

It can be hard to tell your loved ones that they have hurt you. An example of this is when you are dealing with your parents. It can be difficult to express to them how they make you feel or how they have hurt you. Perhaps you don't think you can handle disappointment or conflict with your loved ones and resolve it positively. If you don't have trust in people generally because you have been taken advantage of or mistreated in the past, you may not want to open up about how you feel.

The way you were raised affects how you handle your emotions. As a child, if you are told that your emotions and opinions are not important, then you become very good at hiding them. Experiencing criticism or ridicule when expressing emotion as a child will have a negative effect on you as an adult and you'll be less likely to want to show your emotions. Some adults frown upon any emotional outburst a child may have; this conditions that child to suppress all their emotions, whether good or bad.

The Effects of Suppressing Your Emotions

Think of your emotions like a balloon and, every time you don't let them out, the balloon gets bigger. The more you suppress, the bigger the balloon gets, until one day, it pops. On that day you will have no control over who those suppressed emotions land on. Holding back the expression of your emotions actually intensifies those emotions. Anger is not an emotion that is encouraged, and the expression of it is usually not recommended.

In fact, it is a common expectation to always be calm and not express anger. Unfortunately, the more you clamp down on anger, suppressing it and not addressing it or its root cause, the more it grows. As it intensifies, it will get to the point where you cannot suppress it and it will rush forth, sometimes onto someone who is completely innocent and has nothing to do with why you were angry in the first place.

In order to maintain healthy relationships at home and at work, you need to maintain clear channels of communication. These channels assist in a resolution when there is a conflict. When you suppress your emotions, you are hindering clear communication. The people around you won't know what issues or challenges you're having. Suppressing your emotions and not communicating them effectively with those around you may cause resentment and feelings of anger.

When your communication is so disrupted you are compromising relationships with your loved ones instead of being open and honest about how you feel, this avoidance will make your loved one feel shunned and rejected by you. Without even noticing it, you may begin to avoid people who trigger certain emotions within you and jeopardize relationships you don't want to lose. Eventually you will lose touch with your own feelings and have a harder time introspecting to discern how you feel.

You want to be strong for your loved ones, but they feel the same for you. They don't mind carrying any burdens as long as they are helping you to be okay. If you are hiding your feelings, people who truly know you are able to recognize when something is off about you. When you constantly distract them, they may lose confidence in your relationship and they may question if they are truly valuable to your life.

There is a risk of early death linked to emotional suppression. Stress can affect the physical body and lead to chronic issues such as high blood pressure, heart disease, insomnia, and diabetes. Suppressing your emotions can lead to tension and stress, which may cause any one of the above illnesses. If these emotions continue to be suppressed, this can severely curtail your longevity and negatively affect your long-term health.

TOXIC POSITIVITY AND LETTING IT GO

"Toxic positivity involves dismissing negative emotions and responding to distress with false reassurances rather than empathy. It comes from feeling uncomfortable with negative emotions" (Princing, 2021). Although it may come from a good place, toxic positivity may leave you feeling alienated and disconnected. Life is full of ups and downs; bad things are bound to happen in your life. Sayings like, "Everything happens for a reason" or "t was meant to be" are shallow and offer a false reassurance.

It sounds counterintuitive to put *toxic* and *positivity* in the same sentence next to one another. Toxic positivity can come across as if you have no empathy or compassion for someone else's suffering when responding to their crises. Instead of affirming it as negative emotions or experiences, toxic positivity emanates from an inconsiderable place within you. Toxic positivity often rears its ugly head when you don't know how to respond to a difficult situation. The intention is never bad.

When faced with uncomfortable topics, it is not easy to face or address them in a way that is appropriate. Sometimes we mess up. Messing up is normal, but you should be aware of the kind of responses you give when someone is confiding in you. Toxic positivity tries to make someone feel better about the situation but instead pushes them away and shuts them down. You may want to give reassurance instead of listening to the difficult situation your loved one is going through.

Toxic positivity can have a negative impact on your relationships in such a way that people may begin to think that you are fake or relate to them only on a surface level. Even if you sympathize and truly feel bad for others, toxic positivity can misrepresent this concern. When you have children and a toxic positivity is present in your relationship, it can affect them negatively. When you keep telling them that they're okay and everything is fine then they learn that their negative emotions shouldn't come to the surface and they will begin to suppress them.

When you force positivity, it may not necessarily be because of the situation that is in front of you but rather due to your own previous misfortune. You won't be too enthusiastic to face your own negative emotions, but putting a positivity plaster on your feelings has the opposite effect you intend and can seriously damage your mental health. Avoiding your negative emotions simply makes you feel worse as time goes on.

To let go of a toxic positivity one must accept all emotions as they are and when they come. To be authentic is to be able to sit in your feelings when they arise, whether they are positive or negative. When you are feeling angry or sad, it is okay to remain in that state for a little while before trying to transition to a more positive place. True positivity does not mean you ignore your negative emotions. The more you run from your emotions, the more they will haunt you, until you put them to bed.

FIGHT OR FLIGHT

No matter how evolved we become or how civilized we think we are, at our very core we are animals. A psychological reaction that every person has in the face of a situation that is dangerous or threatening is the fight or flight response. This response prepares the body to either fight the threat or run from it by fleeing. The fight or flight response is an evolutionary adaptation in order to increase our chances of survival when we are facing danger. In a person who has an anxiety disorder or any kind of mental disorder, then the fight or flight response may be activated more frequently, more intensely, or at the wrong time.

When the fight or flight response is activated, there are psychological effects that will lead to physical effects in the body.

- **Eyes**: The pupils will dilate in order to allow more light in. This is done in order to improve vision to see your surroundings better.
- **Skin**: Blood flow to the skin will be reduced, creating either pale or flushed skin. The priority of blood will be to flow to essential body parts such as

the muscles, in case the person may need to fight or flee.

- **Heart**: Coronary blood vessels will relax and dilate to allow more blood flow and increase the heart rate. As more blood is carried to the heart, it will become more energized and oxygenated.
- **Lungs**: The bronchi will dilate, increasing the respiration rate. The blood will be further oxygenated.
- **Circulation**: While the blood vessels serving the digestion will constrict, the ones responsible for the muscles will dilate. The skeletal muscles will be prioritized in terms of receiving oxygen, as well as the brain.
- **Liver**: More glycogen will be converted to glucose in order to have a higher availability of glucose for the brain and skeletal muscles.

When you're feeling scared, your body will trigger this response. The threat may be real or it could just be something that is perceived as a threat, even when it is not one. The fight or flight response is instinctual. As soon as our bodies feel the sensations related to stress, this response is triggered. Automatically, all other higher thinking will be shut down. In these moments, a person will not think about anything, and when it comes to reasoning ability, that is severely curtailed as well.

When adrenaline is released, coupled with other stress hormones, your heart will beat faster, your breathing will be faster, and your body will release extra sugars in preparation for a fight or a run. Have you ever felt really scared? In those moments, how did your body feel? These reactions, whether you realized it or not, were your body's way of preparing you to survive the situation.

The fight or flight response is still very relevant today, as we can still face dangers in our environment. Sometimes because the threat is perceived and not real, we need to be aware of our fight or flight response. A majority of the situations you may find yourself in are not going to allow you to fight or flee. What are you going to do when it is not appropriate to fight or to run away?

Processing the Fight or Flight Response

When the fight or flight response has been triggered, you may need to take some time to think about why you feel this way. What is causing these intense feelings that requires you to want to get physical or run away? It is important to try to get to the root cause of the trigger at a later time, but in the moment the best thing to do is the following:

1. **Remove yourself from the situation:** If you find yourself in a situation where this response is triggered, that means your mind is perceiving a threat and your body will respond accordingly. It is difficult to switch off the response; therefore, to calm

yourself down, you should put as much distance between you and the situation as possible.

2. **No actions:** Once you have removed yourself from the triggering situation, it is best to retire to a safe and peaceful environment where you can take some deep breaths and relax. When the fight or flight response is triggered, it is important not to do or say anything until you are back to a normal mindset.

3. **Work it out:** In order to allow your body to work through the released chemicals, it may be beneficial to partake in some cardio, exercise, or brisk activity. The hormones that we released were helping you to survive by fighting for your life or running for your life, so you need some vigorous activity to make them go away. The suggested activities also reduce endorphins that will make you feel safe and happy. Leaving the hormones in your body will make you more anxious.

4. **Face your problems afterward:** When your body is back to normal, then you can attempt to face the issue and solve the problem at hand.

RELEASE THE BUILDUP

There is a need to express your negative emotions or to work through them in order to enjoy the present moment and not to be hindered by their effects. By doing this you are making space for positive emotions, such as the feeling of success and being fulfilled. Being able to express your negative emotions is necessary if you want to cope with the stress of daily life.

Emotions and stress may be intangible things, but they show up in a physical way if you do not deal with them. Chronic stress can affect your neck, face, shoulders, lungs, your heart, and muscles. If you are stressed and have no effective way to release your stress or negative emotions, it will negatively affect your body and can even cause chronic conditions such as heart disease and high blood pressure.

In order to avoid the negative health implications, you need to release your emotional buildup before you explode. When you take on too much it can also affect your mental health, and take you to a place where you have a mental breakdown. You may not have a lot of control over the kind of stress or the negative emotions that enter your life, but you do have control over how you cope with it.

Whether the emotion is frustration, anger, or anxiety, there are healthy ways you can manage how you feel and deal with the emotions in a constructive manner.

Breathe

When you go into fight or flight mode, you tend to take quicker and shallower breaths. This frantic breathing is fueling this response and it doesn't allow you to reason in the moment. Do not overlook the power of controlling your breathing when you need to release any kind of negative emotion. To combat this feeling, take control of your breathing and you will feel your body instantly relax.

The goal is to breathe from your diaphragm and not from your chest. Sit on a chair or any comfortable place. Allow your shoulders and neck to unwind and relax. Take a slow deep breath through your nose until your lungs fill; exhale slowly through your mouth. Repeat this breathing exercise for as long as you need in order to calm yourself.

What can further make your breathing exercises effective is to visualize that release of the negative emotion as you are exhaling. You breathe in the current situation and then you release it with your exhale. Remind yourself that this feeling is temporary, much like all feelings. This too shall pass.

Do Something Positive

You can spiral into a negative space when you are struggling to release a negative emotion. You can feel like all there is is negativity and that you will never get through the emotions. Perhaps you have held onto them for so long that you don't know how to let go of the negativity. Try to do something positive, either for yourself or for someone else in your life. Trying to be positive when you're in a bad space can shift your mindset.

When you do something positive, you are introducing your positive emotions into your mind. These feel-good sensations remind you that the negative ones are fleeting and that you have control over what you do. It is also very satisfying to be the source of something good. Humor is also a good way to diffuse negative emotion; try to find the humor in a frustrating situation. If you laugh, the scenario has changed and some positivity is present.

Stretch

All the negative emotion and stress we feel is carried in our joints and muscles. In order to release the stress from our physical bodies, we can take part in activities that discharge these emotions and release the tension. Taking a brisk walk or dancing may allow your body to stretch out the tension. An activity that is even more effective is yoga.

To reconnect your mind with your intuitive side, you should try to observe where your body is feeling the tension. Where are you tight? If your mind is closed then your body is also closed. When you are stretching, you can visualize all the tension and stress being relieved from your muscles. As your body loosens up, imagine it opening itself up to receive more positive experiences.

Work Out

Getting your body moving in such a way that your blood is rushing through your body and you are sweating creates a physical release for negative emotions. As you are working out, you may be soothing back pain or stiff muscles and joints. Feel-good hormones are released via this vigorous activity. Exercise is beneficial to reducing depression, anxiety, and negative thoughts.

Readjust Your Perspective

When bad things happen and you have been suppressing your emotions or you have some kind of emotional buildup, it can skew your perspective on what is happening. High-stress situations have the ability to warp your perception of what is real. Everybody has their bad days; when all your stress and negative emotions are at a peak, it can feel like the world is out to get you, but I guarantee you will not feel like that the next day.

When you get a good night's sleep your brain is able to reset and cope better with negative emotions. If you become sleep-deprived you may develop an inability to regulate your emotions, which will exacerbate emotional distress. Making sure you rest your mind and your body will allow you to recover mentally and physically from negative emotions. Sleep is necessary for your overall good health and allows you to have a stable emotional state in order to deal with negative emotions.

Visualize

Using positive and happy thoughts when you are in a negative space can calm your mind and body. Painting a mental picture of something that calms you can help you diffuse boiling tension in the moment. The things you visualize do not have to be things you have done or places you have been to; visualizations can be anything that you want them to be, whether real or aspirational.

Think of a place that makes you feel calm and safe. It can be a babbling brook that you saw during a picnic when you were camping last month, or it can be a white, sandy beach that you would like to see on vacation with your family. Immerse yourself in this place that you have gone to in your mind; what do you see? What do you hear? What do you feel while you are there? This serene and peaceful state should be saved in your mind for whenever you feel your anxiety beginning to rise.

Vent

When you are faced with negative emotions, sometimes it is beneficial to talk with a trusted loved one about how you feel. Venting to your support system may not solve the problem, but it will make you feel better because you have expressed how you feel. It may feel refreshing, as if you have a weight lifted off your shoulders.

Closing yourself off from those people who care about you is not a good thing to do as you are adding to your emotional buildup. Venting to a good friend in times of stress can aid in the reduction of cortisol, which is a hormone that is released during times of stress. There is a reason why you are not walking around the earth on your own; lean on your loved ones for support so that you can process your emotions and express yourself when you are faced with a tough situation.

CHANNEL THE NEGATIVE

Negative emotions do not only have to serve as a hindrance in your life, but they can also drive you to action that benefits you. Instead of feeling pity for yourself, perhaps you can channel your negative emotion and turn it into positive action. When you have understood how you feel and identified why you feel that way, you can move onto using those emotions for good.

Following stress and negative emotion, find a time to sit with a pen and paper to write down what your intentions are. It sounds simple, but doing it can refine your clarity on what your goals are. Negative emotions can cloud your judgment and make you feel demotivated. Writing down your intentions or what you are committed to can help you refocus your mind when it is muddled by negativity.

Draw out a plan on how you will implement these intentions. What action is necessary in order to make your intentions a reality? Keeping your intentions as intentions and failing to draw out a plan on how they are supposed to come to fruition will trap them into being ideas on a piece of paper. Try to figure out what the details are and write them down.

Go public with your intentions and action plan. Letting people know what your intentions are and how you intend on going about making them happen may assist in making sure you follow through. When no one knows what the intentions are or how we plan to carry them out, we are not under any pressure to comply. No one will encourage you or ask you how far you are with your plans if they don't know about them. This external expectation and encouragement can help remotivate you during dark days.

ACT

This chapter has provided you with multiple ideas and avenues that you can use in order to process and release stress and negative emotions. What works for me may not necessarily work for you. You have to customize this information in order to customize your experience. Create some kind of relief plan that you can follow every time you find yourself experiencing emotional turmoil. Remember that, even when you are experiencing negative emotions, it doesn't have to end as a negative experience.

Getting comfortable with regulating and processing your emotions allows you peace and happiness. You will no longer dread being in certain scenarios because you have the skills needed in order to cope in a healthy manner. You can now move forward in your journey of emotional mastery and explore why you think the way you do.

4

THOUGHTS AND FEELINGS

The degree of one's emotions varies inversely with one's knowledge of the facts.

— BERTRAND RUSSELL

By this point, you have understood that your emotions are tools that you can use in order to learn more about yourself. You are working toward not suppressing how you feel, even if those emotions are negative. You now understand that emotions are temporary and that they do not define who you are. The previous chapter dealt with the stigma of facing and expressing your emotions as well as avoiding toxic positivity. In this chapter we will discuss how your thoughts as a black woman may affect your emotion.

Your thoughts may actually be the cause of your negative emotions. It is possible that your thoughts are influenced by past experiences and are therefore misleading and not based on fact. Your core beliefs about the world may be hindering you from being emotionally stable. By the end of this chapter, you should be able to analyze your thoughts and decipher if they are based on fact or if there is another way to look at the situation. You need to be able to understand and unpack why your thoughts are making you feel bad.

THOUGHTS CREATE REALITY

The thoughts you have in your mind will create the experiences you have. What you entertain in your mind and where you let your thoughts go will directly influence your emotions on a daily basis, your behavior, and your experiences. It can be assumed that you are what you think. Your thoughts trigger certain emotions, which will influence what actions you take.

If you get stuck in a thought cycle that depicts you as a failure, you will feel discouraged and like you don't matter. Your posture will reflect these feelings and you may begin to feel aches in your shoulders and back. This might make you feel demotivated and want to remain in bed. Staying in bed for long periods of time instead of chasing your dreams will do nothing to change your situation.

Conversely, if you entertain thoughts that are empowering, you are likely to feel confident, motivated, and in a positive mindset. Your posture will be erect, your shoulders squared, and your head held high. You are more likely to jump out of bed and get right into the actions of the day. When you are energized by your thoughts, you become relentless at achieving your goals. The quality and content of your thoughts will trigger what emotions you feel.

DISTORTION

The way you think directly influences what you believe. The thought patterns that you have developed through your life fuel what you believe about your life and the world. If you think something over and over, it can create a habit. This means you will keep thinking the same thoughts that will create the same kind of emotions, which will lead to you taking the same actions and reliving the same experiences.

To break the pattern, you need to discern where your thoughts are not factual or distorted by past experience. "Anyone can experience cognitive distortion, which the American Psychological Association defines as 'faulty or inaccurate thinking, perception or belief.' Negativity is often the defining characteristic" (UPMC HealthBeat, 2021).

Cognitive distortion is not bad if it is not a part of your thought patterns.

When cognitive distortion is intertwined with your daily thinking patterns, it will interfere with your life and the relationships you have. Cognitive distortion may lead to depression, chronic anxiety, behavioral issues, and addiction. You may be affected by cognitive distortions without being aware of it. The following scenarios outline the most common cognitive distortions that you can fall victim to.

Discounting the Positive

The thinking pattern of a person who constantly discounts the positive degrades a person's self-esteem and pride. This often leads to anxiety. For example, when you receive an award at your workplace, you may refuse to take credit and make excuses, such as pointing out that they gave you the award because you're a woman or that you're black. You may tend to focus on one negative piece of feedback instead of multiple positive ones.

Being Caught Up in Catastrophic Thinking

With this kind of thinking, you tend to expect the worst at all times, in every situation. If you are caught up in this kind of thinking, it can be influenced by and lead to various mental health issues, such as anxiety disorders and depression. Catastrophic thinking negatively affects relationships because the person engaging in this type of thinking may view things as pointless. For example, you might always think somebody died if you get a call from a relative, or think that your partner is leaving you every time they want to talk about serious topics.

Mislabeling

If you often find yourself labeling others or yourself with negative labels, then you may be trapped in this thinking pattern. When you are labeling someone or yourself it is usually based on one past event or previous behavior. Thinking that you are lazy because you can't wake up on time or that your child is a naughty because they got into your makeup last month is mislabeling; the consequence is that it can damage how you view others and yourself. This may have a similar effect to depression on your mind.

Reasoning Based on Emotions

When you base your thoughts on feelings, it can be harmful to you and those around you. If you feel something, it doesn't mean it is a fact. For example, you may feel like your child is being disrespectful when they correct your behavior, or think you are a bad friend because you feel like one. Reasoning based on emotions will likely lead to irrational judgments and decision-making that may cause behavioral issues such as eating disorders.

Jumping to Conclusions

Failing to ask what another person is thinking and then subsequently basing your decisions on what you believe they are thinking will lead to you jumping to conclusions. Making assumptions and filling in the gaps by thinking you know what someone is thinking is mind reading; fortune-telling is thinking that you can predict the future. Thinking that there is no point in learning how to cook because everyone in your family is a bad cook or assuming your partner doesn't love you because they were late for dinner is jumping to conclusions.

Mentally Filtering

If you have a negative filter on your life, then you will not notice or give attention to anything positive that happens. You may see yourself, your past, current, and future, through this negative lens. This means no matter what achievements you get or the number of good things that happen in your life, you will be focusing only on the negative. For example, if you get a promotion at work, you won't be able to celebrate it because you are focusing on the fact that you dropped out of university and you'd be much further ahead in your career if you hadn't.

Personalization

Taking things too personally might trap you in a negative place. Personalization is where you may blame yourself for things that are out of your control. For example, you may think you are a bad mother because you gave birth via cesarean section instead of naturally. This kind of thinking is flawed because giving birth is a situation that is out of everyone's hands. You may feel attacked because you may falsely assume things that people say are directed to you; you may feel constantly excluded and compare yourself to others often.

Overgeneralization

If you have failed once at something it doesn't mean that you will fail again. Those who overgeneralize may take their experience and apply it to every other event they face in their life. For example, if you fail one module you may think there is no point taking it again or trying another one, because you are just agreeing to keep failing. This thinking pattern will soil your view of the world and damage your self-esteem.

Shoulds

Keeping a list of what should and shouldn't be done in terms of people's behavior, or putting blame on others or yourself for failing to do what should have been done or said, is not a healthy thought pattern. If this is something you constantly do, you are inevitably going to experience increased anxiety and stress. Focusing on what should have been will take away the joys happening in the present. For example, if you serve a delicious meal yet you burned the green beans, you won't be able to enjoy the fact that you gave your family an enjoyable meal because you're focusing on the fact that the green beans should have been perfect.

Polarized Thoughts

This thinking pattern encourages extremes. There is good and there is bad, and nothing in between. In your mind, you don't leave room for balanced outcomes or perspectives; there is only failure or success. This kind of thinking can make you feel more stressed out because there is so much pressure to succeed and not fail.

CORE BELIEFS

A person's core beliefs are the ideas they believe about the world, others, and themselves; those ideas influence how they think. Core beliefs are kind of like a filter, or a lens, through which you view life and every situation that you're in. This is why you find that people who experience the same thing, but have different core beliefs, end up thinking and behaving differently. Core beliefs can be inaccurate but still have the same effect on a person; the way that a person sees the world will still be shaped by this erroneous core belief.

Harmful Core Beliefs

You may believe that you are helpless; as a core belief this brings about statements such as 'I'm trapped'; 'I'm weak'; or 'I'm a loser'. You might believe that you are unlovable; this evokes statements such as 'I am going to be alone forever'; and 'Nobody likes me.' Core beliefs that are based on feelings of worthlessness may bring about statements such as, 'I'm worthless'; 'I don't deserve to live'; or 'I'm bad.' If a person has a core belief that there is external danger everywhere they may think, 'No one can be trusted'; 'Nothing ever goes right'; and 'The world is a dangerous place.'

There are interpersonal and mental health consequences if someone carries harmful core beliefs. You may have difficulty trusting others, experience excessive jealousy, become a people-pleaser, feel inadequate in relationships, or become overly aggressive. This may lead to anxiety, low self-esteem, substance abuse, an inability to cope with stress, and depression. Luckily, your core beliefs are not something that you are born with and can be unlearned.

Core beliefs are usually formed in your childhood or during a traumatic period that you experience in your adulthood. Although your core beliefs can be changed, they are inflexible, and even if you observe or experience information that contradicts them, that information is often ignored. Core beliefs that are harmful or negative are not always true, even if you feel that they are.

Identifying Harmful Core Beliefs

Have you had a negative experience in your life that shaped a harmful core belief? You have to first identify your core beliefs before you can begin doing the work to change them. Ask yourself why you have low self-esteem; why do you think you are not worthy? Take time to reflect on your negative experiences and then ponder the following question and write down your answers.

1. How did these experiences make me feel inadequate? What did the experience make me think was wrong with me?
2. Are there specific memories that bring negative thoughts about myself to mind?
3. When I recall these memories, what do I think they say about me as a person?
4. Is there someone in my life I can link to how I feel about myself?
5. Do they describe me in a certain way?
6. What words do they use?
7. What does it say about me as a person if they treat me that way?

Changing Harmful Core Beliefs

Choose a core belief that you would like to work on. You have to try to give yourself balanced core beliefs instead of trying to erase the negative ones. You have to analyze if this belief has seeped into your life and find out what evidence you have based this belief on. Ask yourself:

- Do I have current problems based on this belief?
- Do I condemn myself because I may be struggling to cope on my own and may need help?
- Do I condemn myself for past mistakes?
- Do I condemn myself for my weaknesses?
- Do I condemn myself based on my personality or physical appearance?

- Do I base my worth on how I compare to others?
- Do I base my worth on how others treat me?
- Do I base my worth on how others behave?
- Have I lost something that is tied to my self-worth?

After finding the evidence that the beliefs are based on, it is time to assess if this evidence is credible or false. Think of yourself like a lawyer who is cross-examining a witness in order to decipher the veracity of the evidence they have given. Can you see this evidence from a different perspective where there are other explanations for the evidence? Can you interpret the evidence in different ways where you are not condemning yourself?

After considering different ways to view your evidence, you can probably notice that you have judged yourself too harshly. This is inaccurate and unfair evidence that you used to base the negative view of yourself on. It is difficult to do this exercise at first, but the more you do it the easier it becomes. Based on this new perspective of yourself, start to develop new core beliefs.

ARE MY THOUGHTS TRUE?

If you have realized that your thoughts may be holding you back, you may have to begin seriously questioning them. Analyze these thoughts; sometimes you believe something for so long that it may feel like it's the truth. Thinking something does not make it true for you or anyone else. Every time you feel a thought may be affecting you negatively, ask yourself:

- Is this thought true?
- In this scenario, do I have all the facts?
- How do I know that this thought is true?
- Is there another perspective I can look at this? What might it be?
- Is there another explanation or a way to think differently?

CATCH THOSE THOUGHTS BEFORE THEY AFFECT YOU

How do you know that the thought is a negative one? What are the characteristics of a negative thought? They can be intrusive and take over your mind even if you don't want them to; sometimes they can be automatic, where they enter your mind without any prompting. These thoughts may be very believable, even though they are not true, as well as being distorted and unhelpful. They can make it difficult for you to go after what you want and cripple you. It is important to catch negative thoughts as they arise so that you can stop the pattern.

1. Think about and identify your cognitive distortions. Earlier in the chapter, there was a discussion centered around cognitive distortion. Go through

them and see which ones correspond with your thoughts. Keeping a journal helps in this regard.

2. Challenging negative thoughts is important because we have already established that just because you feel something is true, doesn't make it so. Ask yourself if your thoughts are true? Have you checked the facts?

3. There is no harsher critic than yourself. We judge ourselves constantly; we are so hard on ourselves. The way we speak to our friends and family is not the same way we speak to ourselves. Notice the cognitive distortions that you have identified and give yourself the advice you would give to your good friend. Use a more compassionate and kind tone for any self-talk that you give yourself. It is unhelpful to be unnecessarily hard on ourselves or inflict abuse on ourselves with harsh self-talk. Lead with love and compassion.

4. Seek the help and support of a trusted loved one in order to challenge your cognitive distortions. Getting another perspective may help you to shift your perspective and see things from a different angle. This may lighten your thoughts and reduce anxiety, stress, and depression.

5. Have you gained any benefits from your cognitive distortions? Or would you benefit from challenging them? Answering this will open your eyes to the pros and cons of your current perspective and guide you on whether you should change it or keep it.

TRACK YOUR THOUGHTS

For one week, take time to write down the thoughts you have every day. Challenge each thought by finding some evidence for those thoughts as well as counter-evidence for each unhelpful thought. This will slowly become a habit and you will learn that not all the things you believe to be true, are actually true. Once you master this skill, you will not be controlled by your cognitive distortions and will be able to objectively challenge any negative thought that enters your mind instead of blindly accepting it.

After reining in your negative thoughts, you will need to learn how to be mindful. Emotional self-care and growth is easily achieved if you apply effort to being mindful. This sounds strange if it is a term that is foreign to you. As a black woman, mindfulness may be the key that unlocks all your current frustrations and mental blocks. The next chapter will unpack how exactly mindfulness is a big part of emotional self-care and growth.

5

MINDFULNESS, AWARENESS, AND FOCUS

What you pay attention to grows. If your attention is attracted to negative situations and emotions, then they will grow in your awareness.

— DEEPAK CHOPRA

Mindfulness is a term that has gained fame over the past few years. Perhaps due to the strained and traumatic events that the world has suffered through recently, people recognize that it is important to gain some kind of inner peace. When you are able to control what you give attention to, you have the power to control what affects you. Being mindful, aware, and focused will take you one step closer to mastering your emotions.

There is so much noise in the world. Social media has given everyone a platform to share their opinion, even if that opinion is spewing hate. There are opinions on who is hot and who is not, opinions that may subtly oppress the black woman. If you can take the opportunity to be mindful, you can block out the things that bring you down and realign yourself to what is uplifting and motivating. The resilience that we are known for is easily achieved with mindfulness.

SO, WHAT IS MINDFULNESS?

Before I outline what mindfulness is, perhaps it would be beneficial to briefly state what the benefits might be. You might become even more motivated to be mindful when you are aware of how it can change your life. Mindfulness allows you to take care of your emotional well-being, just like you may go to the gym and eat a balanced diet to take care of your physical body. Mindfulness will keep you centered and grounded while you grow and reach for your dreams; if you establish strong roots then you will be an unshakable force. Being mindful makes you aware of any self-sabotaging behavior; you have an opportunity to address yourself with respect, kindness, and compassion.

After practicing mindfulness, you will become the most authentic version of yourself. Because of this, it will be easier to develop healthy and fulfilling relationships with our loved ones. It will also be easier to recognize toxic relationships and set boundaries for yourself. When you are a safe haven for yourself, you are shutting out the microaggressions that are around you and that you have to deal with on a daily basis, every time you walk out of the door or look at your phone. Your resilience will build from the fact that you rest your emotions within mindfulness.

"Mindfulness is the basic human ability to be fully present, aware of where we are and what we're doing, and not overly reactive or overwhelmed by what's going on around us" (Mindful Staff, 2020). Everyone has had the ability to be mindful. If it is not something that you have been practicing, then it is something that you can learn how to do. Being mindful can assist in the regulation of our emotions; it can also reduce stress, depression, and anxiety. When you're practicing mindfulness, you are able to focus your attention. You can also allow your thoughts and feelings to exist without judging yourself.

Practicing mindfulness can be done in various ways whether you are sitting, standing, walking, or moving. It can be a set time you use every day or short sessions throughout your day. Activities such as yoga can be used in order to practice mindfulness and meditation. Being mindful is not something that is happening in your head because it encompasses your entire body. You have to pay attention to what you are feeling in your body and thinking in your mind. Practicing mindfulness will remove you from a downward spiral if you have been under emotional stress, and put those traumatic events into perspective so that you do not develop cognitive distortions.

Mindful Eating

You can practice mindfulness in your eating by stopping yourself from not partaking in mindless eating. We all do it when we reach for food while scrolling through our phone or chatting to our friends. Take note of what you are eating in order to fuel your body. Do not multitask while you eat. Be present as you eat your food; take note of every bite and pay attention to the taste and texture of the food. Listen to the signals your body is sending about whether or not you are getting full. Being mindful about eating will ensure you are more intentional about what you put on your plate.

Mindful Interactions

It is important to be mindful when you are interacting with those around you. Sometimes we don't really listen to the people around us even when we are in a one-on-one conversation with them. To be mindful during an interaction means observing what the person is doing and remaining present during the conversation. Give them your undivided attention, and also notice how you are feeling during that interaction. When you are more mindful with your relationships you learn to listen carefully and respond without reacting.

Mindful Activities

Sometimes you get up from where you are sitting and walk into another room but, once you get there, you completely forget why you wanted to be there. Has that ever happened to you? Have you ever walked out of your home, locked the door, walked a few steps, and wondered if you locked the door, only for you to go back to check and find that you did lock it? Those things are happening because you are not being mindful when you are engaging in activities. You have multiple opportunities to be mindful in your activities because you do so much in one day.

Instead of rushing through your chores or activities during the day, take the time to perform those various tasks with a heightened awareness. As you clean your home, do not think of anything else but the activity you are doing at that moment; if you are mopping, focus on the actions of the mop going back and forth on the floor. Feel the warmth of the water between your fingers as you wring the mop and watch the suds get disturbed every time you reimmerse the mop in the water.

BE MORE MINDFUL

We have conditioned ourselves to do so much in a short amount of time. As women, we are renowned multitaskers. We can cook a meal while loading the washing machine and watching the news. Imagine how many times your attention is refocused when you are doing all these things at the same time. There is so much room for mistakes when you are not fully focusing on what you are doing. This habit of doing too many things at one time can leave you feeling overworked and frustrated. It is important to learn how to be more mindful in order to live a stress-free life.

Pay attention to what you are doing. You can end up taking longer to complete a task and make more errors when you are multitasking. You may find that you actually finish faster and make less errors when you focus on that one thing. Make it a point to only do one thing at a time and not to begin a new task until you have completed the one you are busy with. Slow things down and savor each step of completing that task. Be intentional and deliberate. Having a healthy focus on your tasks will lessen the feeling of being overwhelmed.

Our minds are almost always traveling at 100 mph thinking about what needs to be done next and how we're going to do it even before we have finished what we are doing now. You are never truly focused in the moment and can fail to notice vital things around you. Focus on the moment. Our generation is so focused on recording everything for our timelines that we cannot focus on and enjoy special moments, or even the small moments in our everyday life. Take note of your five senses and notice what you see, hear, taste, touch, and smell. Focus on the moment and how you feel about it; what thoughts are running through your mind?

Our breathing can either calm us down or keep us rooted in our mindfulness. If ever you feel the need to practice mindfulness in a moment of distress or if you feel your thoughts taking you to an undesirable place, then it can be helpful to use your breathing to be mindful. Taking a deep breath in, holding it for a few seconds, and then slowly exhaling can bring you into the moment and root you in it. Your mind will have to focus on following your breath, and this will make you more conscious of where you are and what is happening. Focus on your breathing and you will automatically be more mindful.

FOCUS

The things that you focus on is where your energy is directed toward and what you will pay more attention to. For example, if you focus on all your failures, your energy will be spent thinking about all the things you have failed at and what you could have done better, and then the idea that you are Ophelia will get bigger and bigger. Focusing on the thoughts and emotions that don't bring you joy and keep you unhappy will further depress you, keeping you in an unhappy and dissatisfied state. You can choose to keep your mind on these unhelpful thoughts or you can decide to focus on more uplifting and positive thoughts.

Sometimes your mind is in the right place but you just can't concentrate on what you are supposed to do. Your focus can be affected by internal and external factors; it can be things that are within your control and those that are out of your control. You need to be able to focus on what will help you further your goals and ambitions. Focus is vital to your success and you should be able to concentrate on what's important so that you don't get in your own way.

IMPROVE FOCUS

No Distractions

Eliminating destruction is key to improving your focus. No matter where we are or what we are doing, there is a persistent stream of information that is coming toward us. Technology has not made it easy to remain focused, as your smartphone serves as a constant distraction. Try to remove everything that can distract you, such as putting your phone in your bag and closing any tabs on your computer that may steal your attention. If you can, it can be helpful to close the door so that people around you can see that you're busy. Schedule a time and place to do a specific task and let others know that they cannot disturb you during this time.

No Multitasking

The previous section has already outlined how multitasking is detrimental to being mindful. Unfortunately, multitasking is also responsible for lower focus, lower productivity, and poor concentration. Focusing on various things while attempting to do one task compromises the quality of all the things you're doing. It may feel like you are being very productive by doing one million things at once, but it is a recipe for disaster. Focus on one task and finish it before beginning another; if you need to take a break, then do so and resume when you are refreshed.

Meditation and Mindfulness

Meditation can be used to become more mindful and you may also practice mindful activities so that you are mentally and emotionally fit and able to focus. When you meditate, your brain is achieving a higher level of calmness, which will lead to a more relaxed body. Our minds are always running through various thoughts at all times; therefore, being able to focus on our breath ensures that we do not get distracted. Breathing is an effective tool that can be used to bring our focus back to what we are doing no matter how many times we get interrupted.

Sleep More

Technology here is an enemy once again because the LED screens from our phones and television screens emit blue light that stimulates the retina and suppresses melatonin secretion. Melatonin is responsible for letting our brains know that sleep is anticipated. It is important to avoid technology toward bedtime so that sleep is not disturbed. Other ways to aid the improvement of sleep include staying well hydrated, exercising earlier in the day, and using breathing or journaling to clear the mind and achieve emotional stability. Ensure that you have a set bedtime schedule that you do not deviate from.

Choose the Moment

Anxiety is caused by worrying about the past or future. Focusing on the present is difficult as the past is not easy to let go of, especially if it includes traumatic events. We are constantly worrying about our future, the future of our families, and where our lives are going. Acknowledge the event and the lessons it came with, then do your best to let it go. Do the same thing with the worry you have for the future. Notice how the anxiety is affecting your body and then let it go. Choose to focus on the moment because your mind will go where you choose to place your focus.

Be in Nature

As human beings, we can forget that we are animals simply because we have evolved so much. Our natural habitat is in nature and not in the buildings and skyscrapers. Taking a walk in a garden or doing some gardening can increase your concentration and leave you feeling refreshed. If you can't go to nature, you can bring nature to you by having plants in your office space and at home. They will improve the air quality and increase satisfaction and productivity.

Brain Training

You can take part in brain training activities that will enhance your concentration. This includes brain training games that will assist in boosting your short-term and working memory. Games such as chess and sudoku can assist in improving your problem-solving and processing skills. There are even brain-stimulating video games that you can play that will improve your cognitive abilities. This will inevitably improve your focus and you will be able to concentrate better. You can also train your brain with meditation, which will improve your focus as well.

BUILDING SERENITY

Serenity is the state of being serene, but what is it to be serene? As defined by the Merriam-Webster Dictionary (n.d.), being serene is "utter calmness, or quietude." What would it take for you to feel serene and live in a continuous state of serenity? Instead of remaining in a state of stress and emotional imbalance, building serenity will allow you to savor feelings of peace and calm in your life.

You have to be able to control the responses you give to the things that life throws at you. It is obvious that you can't control life, and you also can't control other people and how they treat you. The only thing that you are in control of is your environment and your responses. When you are able to control your responses, you will no longer feel overwhelmed by feelings of anxiety; these feelings will become manageable and peace will be the default setting in your life. To build serenity in your life, there are seven habits that you need to take part in:

1. What you do when you wake up first thing in the morning is what will set the tone for the rest of your day. Incorporate a morning ritual that will calm you and settle your emotions; the earlier you get up, the better. Staying in bed for an extended period of time is tempting but it creates a sense of chaos in your morning, as you will be rushing to leave your house on time and risk being late for school or work. If one thing goes wrong it can derail you completely. Mornings are quite serene and if you wake up early you can exercise or meditate and enjoy their peaceful nature.

2. Every time you are faced with stress you react in a certain way. Perhaps you have unhealthy coping mechanisms that help you get through stressful situations. For example, a smoker will tend to smoke more when they are under stress, and someone who leans on alcohol will drink more. Notice the behaviors you turn to when you come under stress: Do you feel overwhelmed, do you distract yourself and run from the situation, or do you face the stress head on?

3. If you haven't been responding to stress in a healthy way, it is now time to respond in a healthier way. You know all the ways to respond that are not helpful or beneficial. Replace them with an activity that will bring you peace. For example, instead of going outside and smoking a

cigarette, perhaps make a cup of tea or meditate for five minutes.

4. Sometimes the reason why we feel attacked is because we take everything personally. Luckily, the truth of the matter is that most things are not about you or directed at you. You are probably not the reason that someone is in a bad mood. Do not take everything so personally and you will likely feel more at peace.

5. If you read a lot of self-help books, you may know that a lot of them emphasize gratitude. This is because keeping track of the things you are grateful for when you are going through a challenging time will put things into perspective. You will feel better when you think about all the things that you are grateful for. Gratitude gives you the good vibes needed to tackle any issues that hinder your progress in life.

6. Doing one thing at a time also provides you peace and serenity in your life as your mind is not cluttered by multitasking.

7. I live a simple life that is devoid of clutter. If your environment is filled with too many things, you won't be able to think clearly. This is why open spaces are so refreshing. If there is a lot of noise around you, then you need to reduce this noise and keep sound levels at a peaceful tone. Get rid of things that are cluttering your space and your life.

MINDFULNESS EXERCISES

- **Mindful observation:** This exercise involves watching an object in your immediate environment and concentrating on it. Explore its formation, every corner and curve, and try to connect with its energy and purpose.
- **Mindful awareness:** This exercise should give you added appreciation of daily tasks. Take a task that you do every day, such as making a cup of coffee, and really immerse yourself in it. Every time something hits your senses, be grateful; when you smell the aroma of the coffee, appreciate how fortunate you are that you have a good cup of coffee to enjoy.
- **Mindful listening:** With this exercise you are learning the ability to listen from a neutral perspective without any preconceptions. Close your eyes and listen to some music. Keep your mind open, do not be hindered by the artist or genre, and allow yourself to get lost in the instruments, the voices.
- **Mindful appreciation:** Notice a few things in your life that go unappreciated, such as the electricity in your home or the running water in your tap. List five things and try to explore how they came about, what keeps them going, and how they relate to everything else around you, to encourage yourself to appreciate them.

Life is not always easy, and that is something that you have to learn how to cope with. Mindfulness allows you to create some kind of peace in your life, but sometimes you can still become overwhelmed by your emotions. If you don't develop the skill of coping with bad feelings, you will easily become suffocated by them. The next chapter will talk about how to face bad feelings when they overwhelm you.

6

FACING BAD FEELINGS

If you don't think your anxiety, depression, sadness and stress impact your physical health, think again. All of these emotions trigger chemical reactions in your body, which can lead to inflammation and a weakened immune system. Learn how to cope, sweet friend. There will always be dark days.

— KRIS CARR

L ife comes with challenges. Those challenges may come with bad emotions that make you feel worse about yourself. Feeling bad is normal, but it is not often that we want to find out why we are feeling bad. Are your thoughts responsible for your bad feelings or do they emanate from a physical need that has not been attended to? Perhaps it is your environment that is creating these bad feelings. What can you do to make yourself feel better or differently?

Facing your bad feelings is inherent in emotional self-care. It has been established that your feelings serve as messengers to alert you of something that is wrong. In order to truly understand why you are feeling bad you will have to explore and sit with these bad feelings. The more you ignore them the bigger they will get, until they completely consume you and wreak havoc on your mental health. But to feel good emotionally and physically you have to face your emotions, even when they are not desirable.

DEPRESSION

"A negative affective state, ranging from unhappiness and discontent to an extreme feeling of sadness, pessimism, and despondency, that interferes with daily life" (American Psychological Association, 2014). If the depression is left untreated it can completely derail your life. And you need to constantly acknowledge and express yourself when it comes to your negative thoughts and feelings. In order to avoid feeling depressed, you can do so many different things to lessen the symptoms of depression.

If you want to empower yourself to deal with your depression then you should accept yourself and be open and loving to where you are emotionally. Do not force yourself to be happy; if you need to wallow, then wallow. Sit on your feelings then journal about them. Understand that just because you had an off day today doesn't mean you will have the same type of day tomorrow. If your depressed voice is leading you in one direction, go in the opposite direction. Create a routine that will make you feel in control; this routine should be flexible, but include key aspects such as working out and meditation in the morning and journaling or blogging in the evening.

The best thing to do when you're in a funk is to do something you like. Get immersed in the enjoyment and enjoy every moment. Likewise with your loved ones; they will improve your mood and get you motivated to tackle your challenges; therefore, spend more time with them when you're feeling depressed. Giving to those who are in need of volunteering will create good-feel vibes that will also spark feelings of gratitude. Meditation will lower stress and keep anxiety and other mental health issues at bay.

When to Seek Help

You can experience episodes of depression more than once in your life. During these episodes, the symptoms will bother you most of the day for consecutive days. Symptoms of depression include:

- Unexplainable back or head aches
- Suicidal thoughts or attempts
- Feeling worthless
- Restlessness, irritability, or agitation
- Unexplained weight loss
- Reduced appetite
- Excessive food cravings
- Always tired, no energy
- Losing interest in activities you previously enjoyed
- Angry outbursts
- Feeling helpless, empty, or sad

If feelings of depression do not abate after speaking to loved ones or doing any of the suggested activities above, you may need medical help. If the symptoms persist consistently for a fortnight, and this is affecting how you live your daily life, it is time to relinquish control to medical professionals. You will feel the impact of depression when you are not able to do things that are a part of your normal day, such as bathing, cleaning your environment, or preparing nutritious meals.

ANGER

Anger is a very strong emotion that is characterized by hostility, tension, and rising frustration emanating from real or perceived injury by another; anger may also emanate from a perceived injustice. The way that you show anger is different to how the next person may express anger. This is an emotion that is difficult to speak about, as we have always been taught that anger is a bad emotion. The truth is that anger itself is not bad, but rather your reaction is what is bad if you can't control yourself in the face of anger.

When you get angry it is usually because you are scared or someone has violated your boundaries. Feelings of anger can also come from your needs failing to be met. Anger is not an emotion you should suppress at all, as this may lead to nervousness and frustration. If it has been suppressed long enough, it can erupt as an uncontrollable rage via acts of aggression. To remain emotionally healthy, you have to embrace feelings of anger and allow compassion to heal your wounds. Facing this bad feeling can be done in this way:

1. **Be aware of how anger manifests.** Anger can either be turned inward or outward. Outward anger includes indignation, belligerence, revenge, detachment, and contempt. Inward anger includes depression, unworthiness, and self-punishment.
2. **How is anger embodied in you?** Take note of your bodily reactions to anger. How did your breathing change? Did tears form in your eyes? Anger manifests differently in each person so it's important to know how it embodies itself in you.
3. **Dig within yourself.** As a response to being hurt, you get angry. But what is this anger protecting you from? What are the feelings you are running from?

4. **Let anger speak to you.** Imagine your anger as a separate entity. If it could talk, what would it say to you? What message would your anger bring?

5. **Do not expect anything.** Letting go of expectations means you are releasing the way you wanted things to happen. Open your mind to consider alternatives.

6. **Be compassionate to yourself.** This is the emotion that will douse your anger and extinguish harsh self-doubt. Being compassionate to yourself will give you practice so that you can be compassionate to others. Self-compassion brings with it love, respect, and care.

7. **Forgiveness.** This is a liberating action that you can choose to make on a daily basis. You must choose to forgive yourself and those around you consistently in order to live a peaceful life.

8. **Don't get attached.** It is difficult to let go of anger, especially if you feel justified. In order to be able to let it go, you should believe and trust that you will be better off without it. We have little control over what others do and even less control over how life unfolds. Trust that letting go will make you better.

9. **Don't fight your anger.** Struggling against it will make your life harder and delay the processing of your emotions. Ask yourself, if you weren't angry, what would you be feeling? Do not shy away from anger; allow yourself to take a good look at it.

Anger Management Exercises

▷ **Beware of Your Triggers**

Things that get under your skin and set you off are described as anger triggers. When you are aware of your triggers, you can control your anger better. Getting ahead of your triggers will ensure they don't make your anger spiral out of control. In order to use your triggers to your advantage you have to first be able to identify them.

- Create a list of triggers and go over it on a daily basis.
- Make the necessary changes to avoid your triggers, within reason.
- Create an action plan for when you come across your triggers.

▷ **Log All Anger Episodes**

Get in the practice of logging your anger episodes. It will make your triggers, patterns, and warning signs more recognizable.

- Describe what was happening before the episode; what was your emotional and physical state?
- Describe the events. What triggered you? What was your reaction?

- Describe your feelings during the episode and how you felt at the apex of your anger. How could you have reacted better in the moment?

ANXIETY

When you sit with stress for too long, it will develop into anxiety. Stress is unavoidable and it will be lurking behind every corner to affect you. You don't have to be overwhelmed by stress. To manage stress and avoid anxiety, try the following activities:

- Time management can help you effectively manage the tasks in your life.
- Be assertive and address your feelings as they arise instead of suppressing or avoiding them.
- Accept that life is beyond your control.
- Try to remain positive at all times.
- Create boundaries and limits; say no when you need to.
- Do not turn to substance abuse to relieve stress.
- Make time for your interests and loved ones.
- Seek professional help if you are not coping.

Reduce the Unknown

Anxiety is essentially the fear of the unknown. If you are caught up in worrying about the future, it can paralyze you with fear. In order to reduce your anxiety about the future, it would be helpful to remove some of the mystery. Try to plan your life so that you are not in the dark about what you need to do to achieve your goals. Ground yourself in the moment by doing some deep breathing exercises and being mindful about your surroundings. Focus on an object and take in its shape and form so that you can come back to the present. Check if you are living in the present and if you are okay.

Anxiety Management Exercises

- What are 10 things that make you feel scared or nervous?
- What are you thinking about when you become scared and nervous?
- Describe which parts are affected by these feelings of nervousness and fear.
- What can you do to soothe yourself the next time you are scared?

GUILT

Guilt can come from doing something that you regret or when you know you've done something that you could've done better. Guilt is a very powerful emotion, and if you begin to feel it then perhaps you should check on your emotional well-being. If you ever feel guilty about anything, take it as a marker to analyze your behavior and see what you can improve instead of taking your guilt as something that holds you back. If your guilt is becoming overwhelming, then there are certain things you can do to lighten the weight.

- Find the reason for your guilt instead of suppressing it, because unresolved guilt will make you feel worse over time.
- Apologize for your role in whatever situation is making you feel guilty, show remorse, and ask for forgiveness. Do not make excuses for your behavior, take responsibility for the mistakes you have made.
- Learn from the mistakes that you have made in the past and explore what you would do differently in the present. Then let it go.

REGRET

Regret and shame are indicators that you may be reliving the past too much. Sometimes ruminating gets the best of us and we end up getting hung up on what we could have done and the feelings of shame that we still experience in the present. The only way to let go of regret and shame is to go through the process of forgiveness. This forgiveness is toward yourself as well as others, so that you can root yourself in the present and stop living in the past.

How to Forgive

"I repeat that. Forgiveness is giving up the hope that what would have, could have, should have happened, in fact... it did not happen. It's accepting the reality of what did happen, and moving on" (Winfrey, 2021). In order to effectively forgive you have to accept what happened, forgive those that hurt you, forgive yourself for your part, and accept how it has all turned out. When you have mastered this process of forgiveness, you will begin to heal and let go of resentment that may be holding you back.

Having the ability to deal with the bad feelings will take you one step further in your emotional mastery and lessen your apprehension in difficult situations. Now you can equip yourself with some tools that will assist you to manage your emotions better in the present. In the next chapter, I will take you through what you need in order to carry out your emotional self-care.

7

EMOTIONAL CARE TOOLS

*Unleash in the right time and place before you explode at the
wrong time and place.*

— OLI ANDERSON

JOURNALING FOR RELEASE

You can use journaling as an incredible life-changing
tool that will help you work through your emotions.
When life keeps happening, it can get messy and loud. You
may not be able to hear your thoughts and can get lost in
everything. Journaling clears your perspective and will
reveal habits, patterns, feelings, and desires that may have

been shrouded in the clutter of life. Use a journal prompt, which are questions that will prompt your writing. You can write as if you are writing someone a letter. There are no set rules on how you should journal or what you should journal about, so feel free to do what feels natural. When you are writing, let the pen do what it wants and enjoy the process.

Keep your thoughts honest so that you can enjoy the full benefits of journaling. Be vulnerable, because it is a safe space where you can unravel and discover the essence of your truth. You don't need to journal once a day, you can keep your journal with you and keep journaling as your day unfolds. Remain consistent with how and when you journal so that it can become a habit in your life. The more you write, the more you will want to write. This can also be your support habit that you turn to when you are feeling emotionally imbalanced.

ART THERAPY FOR RELEASE

Art

Since the mid-1900s, art therapy has been used in addressing various mental health issues. Art can unlock a certain creativity within you that lies beyond words and sentences. Art will relax you and release you from your state of unease. As you are immersed in your art it will boost mindfulness, because you are completely consumed in the activity. Due to the mindfulness of the activity, you may get a chance to break from your ruminating. Activities such as coloring or painting will get you into a flow state that maximizes your mental engagement and increases your focus.

Music

Music is a powerful tool that can have a life-altering effect on your body and emotions. Music that is more upbeat will wake you up and allow you to focus better; it can give you an optimistic view on life. Slower tempo music will allow your mind to unwind while soothing your stress away. As you listen to the slow rhythm and tempo, your muscles will relax and you may even feel the tension leaving your body. In order to relax while you are conscious, you should listen to music that is around 60 bpm, as your brain will synchronize to the alpha brain waves that are caused by the beat.

HOLISTIC TOOLS

A holistic approach to healing means that not only will you focus on the physical body, but also on your wellness and mental health. You have to see yourself as a whole person that has various aspects that are intertwined and cannot be separated from one another. Healing the mind without healing the body is not effective, just like healing the spirit and not healing the mind is not effective. Your spirit is also connected to your body; you cannot divorce the different aspects of yourself from each other; therefore, it is best to heal yourself holistically.

That being said, what you need to do to treat yourself holistically will differ from what the next person needs to do. Due to your life experiences, triggers, and traumas, you may need a variety of treatments that will address your emotional and mental health issues. Someone else might need to address their toxic positivity and develop a healthier view of themselves. How you apply holistic tools is completely subjective and you have to customize the experience for yourself.

Acupressure for Stress

Based on ancient Chinese medicine, acupressure is a massage where pressure is put on certain points of the body that are called acupoints. When pressing on these acupoints, the pressure will relax muscles and improve blood flow. Acupressure can be done at home when you place your finger and apply pressure to various acupoints. Yin Tang, also referred to as a pressure point extra-1, is a pressure point that is located between your eyebrows. This pressure point is said to relieve anxiety and stress.

In order to do acupressure on Yin Tang, find a comfortable place to lay down, sit, or stand. With either your left or your right hand, place your thumb in between your eyebrows at the center. You should make sure that your thumb is on your forehead and not on the top of your nose. Using your thumb, press down firmly on this point and move your thumb, either clockwise or anticlockwise, in circles for up to three minutes. The pressure you apply to this acupoint shouldn't be painful and you can repeat the acupressure until your symptoms ease.

Cryotherapy

This kind of therapy makes a person sit in a cold tank that is at near-freezing temperatures. Research surrounding cryotherapy is fairly new; therefore, the benefits have not been definitively proven. A person will enclose themselves in a cryotherapy booth for up to five minutes in a spa setting and, though it may feel unpleasant in the beginning, you will get used to it with time. The benefits include healing of painful muscles and joints. People with arthritis or with athletic injuries benefit from cryotherapy. This process is also said to promote weight loss as the cold will kick the body into overdrive, making it work hard to remain warm; this is how fat is burned.

Inflammation is how the immune system fights off infections that are attacking the body; unfortunately, the immune system might become overly sensitive, causing chronic inflammation (leading to diabetes, cancer, dementia, and arthritis). Cryotherapy reduces inflammation, which will prevent dementia and cancer. Cryotherapy will assist in mental health issues, such as anxiety and depression, because they too are linked to inflammation. Eczema and migraines are improved by cryotherapy, although not completely cured.

Psychedelic Therapy

This kind of therapy is also called PAP (psychedelic-assisted psychotherapy) and it involves the patient taking into their bodies a substance that is psychedelic and then going into a psychotherapeutic process. You can take substances that are taken from plants such as magic mushrooms, ayahuasca, or peyote; or the substances that are chemical compounds, such as LSD, MDMA, and ketamine. Psychedelic therapy is new in the western world but it has been used in indigenous communities for centuries in order to tackle issues such as addiction and PTSD, as well as mental health issues such as anxiety and depression.

Clinicians require a consultation first, where your medical history and profile is gathered. Exact dosing has not yet been determined, so it will vary from person to person; after consultation, you will be given a dose of the psychedelic, either by injection or by ingesting it. You will be under the supervision of a trained professional. Following ingestion, there will be integration where the patient and the therapist try to decipher the deeper meaning behind the psychedelic hallucinations, if there were any. Only do psychedelic therapy with professionals and avoid self-medicating.

TRE—Tension- and Trauma-Releasing Exercises

TRE is an innovative way to release tension and stress from the body. Trauma is often carried in the body as well, and it can be released through a series of exercises. The nervous system is put in a calmed state by the activation of a natural reflex mechanism which involves vibration and shaking to release tension in the muscles. Because the vibration is activated in a controlled environment, the body is motivated to return to its natural balance. Stress, trauma, and tension have both physical and psychological effects; therefore, you have to deal with how stress affects your mind, and also how it affects your body.

TRE is a self-help tool that you can practice on your own in order to boost your emotional health. The feeling of the vibrations is soothing and pleasant on the body. Unfortunately, you have to deal with the trauma, stress, and tension you experience, as well as give attention to the small irritations that build up every day. The next chapter will be focused on how to manage your everyday stress. Always keep an open mind when you take part in holistic treatments; what will work for you may surprise you.

8

MANAGING DAY BY DAY

I strive, each day, to be kinder to myself, and to value my worth. And I know I'm not alone.

— MAYA ANGELOU

If you don't deal with stress on a daily basis it will pile up and become a bigger issue than it has to be. Health problems can arise from allowing stress-related hormones to flood your body. Depression, hypertension, heart disease, gut health issues, as well as panic attacks could become real problems in your life if you don't deal with stress factors daily.

EFFECTS OF STRESS

Stress is defined as any response that your brain gives to demands. Stress can be good and it can also be bad, depending how intensely it hits you and for how long. Whether you are treating it or not will also have an effect on the way stress affects you. If you have been living with this stress for an extended period of time it is referred to as chronic or toxic stress, and it can be harmful to how the brain and body function. In the United States a survey conducted in 2015 showed that work and money are the leading causes of stress, and this has been the case for almost a decade.

Stress causes chain reactions in your brain because it delivers stress signals to the hypothalamus. That part of the brain communicates with the nervous system so that the person can go into the flight or fight response. If you want to remind yourself of what the response is about, visit chapter 3. In short, the fight or flight response will create physical reactions such as shallow breathing, increased heart rate, and increased doses of adrenaline in the body.

Chronic stress has even more of a damaging effect on the brain because of a backlog of cortisol. Having too much cortisol in the brain can cripple its functioning. These effects can lead to you avoiding social situations with others. Chronic stress can shrink your brain and kill brain cells. Your memory and learning will be negatively affected because chronic stress disadvantages the prefrontal cortex, which is responsible for these things. Your cognitive functioning can be severely curtailed by chronic stress.

Symptoms of Stress

- Insomnia
- Body aches
- Heart palpitations
- Frequent illness
- Loss of libido or sexual ability
- Being nervous and anxious
- Irritability and severe moodiness
- Low self-esteem
- Avoiding others
- Feeling like you have lost control
- Being unable to relax
- Low concentration and inability to focus
- Substance abuse
- Procrastination

STAY CALM

Stress is inherent in every day and there is no way to avoid it. Your best option is to try to deal with it as the days pass so that it doesn't pile up. Depending on who you are and how much you have on your plate, you may break down when placed in stressful situations. Another person will deal with it calmly because they have the mental strength to adjust to the added pressure. If stress is constantly bringing you down, it can have an adverse effect on your self-esteem and confidence. It is a heavy burden to walk around with a weight on your shoulders or knots in your stomach.

As a black woman, you may face stress at home and at the workplace. You may feel like life keeps throwing you curve-balls and you keep striking out. Stress needs to be handled while you are calm, so that you are facing it with a level head. Even when you feel like you are overwhelmed and drowning inside, you have to try to deal with anger, stress, and fear as they occur. Stress is part and parcel of life; try to learn how to deal with it from an early age so that it doesn't affect your well-being as you get older.

When faced with stress, always try to keep a positive attitude just to see that you are able to meet the challenge with an open mind. Use a realistic approach and research how others have overcome the difficult situation that you are in; perhaps when you see how others were able to overcome, it will motivate you to do the same. Always assert your feelings when you're under pressure and avoid being defensive or passive; being aggressive instead of assertive when you are under pressure is not helpful in the situation, as it can lead to poor decision-making. Asserting your emotions allows you to process them quickly to find immediate solutions from a calm standpoint.

SIMPLIFY YOUR LIFE

Not-To-Do List

You have heard of a to-do list but have you heard of a not-to-do list? A to-do list gives you things that you need to focus on and that should be your priority over everything else. A not-to-do list does the same thing by reinforcing where you shouldn't waste your time. No matter what, you should not do these tasks; rather, you should pass them off to somebody else or pay someone to do them. When asked to do them you should simply say no.

Creating this list will easily remove bad habits and tasks that are not a priority from your life. Things that should be on your not-to-do list include things that are distractions, things you can't say no to, bad habits, emotionally draining tasks, low priority tasks, and tasks that fall under another's responsibility. Take some time to create your own list by finding recurring tasks from previous months. Try to identify the tasks that don't add value to your life and those that you can eliminate or outsource. Additionally, you should also look for activities that come with a negative emotion or you procrastinate to perform.

Add the relevant tasks to the not-to-do list and learn to say no when somebody requests that you perform that task. Learning how to say no to yourself is great practice if you struggle to say no to others. Once you've formulated this list, try to stay faithful to it and review it every other week. Your needs and values should come first. When you are clear on what is for you and what is not, your life will become much simpler.

Do, Defer, Delegate, Drop

- Do small tasks that will give you the momentum and motivation to tackle larger tasks. For example, follow up with a client via email, edit that presentation, or schedule that meeting with your boss. Prioritize.
- Defer/Delay anything that may not be urgent. Anything that has just come up is something that does not need to be completed right away. For example, a request from a colleague or a suggestion to do things differently. Neither of those are urgent, or they can be delayed.
- Delegated tasks that can be performed by anybody else; focus on those that are specific to your skill set.
- Remove any tasks that are not beneficial to your progress.

The points above allow you to be more productive by sifting through your tasks and checking if they are worth spending your time on. You decide whether or not something should be done by you, or if it is a task that you should abandon. This will streamline your productivity and allow you to stay focused on what matters to you.

IS YOUR CONTEXT OFF?

Context is necessary in order not to get carried away by negative emotions or stressful situations. It only takes a series of unfortunate events to unravel you emotionally. External stressors can affect our ability to put things into context. The way you handle a situation is directly influenced by how you think. If you have negative thoughts, you are likely to handle the situation from a negative perspective; similarly, if you have positive thoughts, you will handle the situation positively.

Reframe Your Thinking

The word "reframing" means that you identify thoughts that are second nature to you and replace them with balanced ones; cognitive behavioral therapy uses reframing to dismantle any cognitive distortions people get stuck in. To practice reframing your thoughts, you need to identify the cognitive distortions that are affecting you. Then, you must weigh out all the evidence that supports and thwarts this cognitive distortion. Think about the facts and get a balanced idea of what the truth is; be compassionate toward yourself and be accepting and forgiving while practicing self-love. This will allow you to make room for positive feelings and not fall victim to your negative patterns.

Remove the Triggers

▷ Toxic people

It is difficult to have to deal with toxic people on a daily basis. People who tend to suck the life out of you, who have a negative perspective of life and never stop complaining are commonly referred to as toxic, although this is not a medical definition. Traits of a toxic person include dishonesty, someone who loves sowing chaos and conflict, being self-absorbed, manipulative, and prone to inflict emotional abuse. To deal with such people, you need to avoid validating their reality and respectfully disagree while sticking to facts.

The best thing you can do for yourself while you are dealing with toxic people is to always remain calm and not to stoop to their level. Notice how they make you feel and if this feeling is present during all your interactions. Try to address them about their problematic behavior so that they can understand why their behavior is hurtful and unacceptable. You can be compassionate toward them based on whatever issues they may be struggling with, but it is important to put yourself first and walk away from them and the interaction if it is affecting you mentally and emotionally. Limit your interactions with them and do not make yourself available to their toxicity.

▷ Toxic Overload

The world is full of toxic situations and people. You need to know how to clear out the clutter, remove distraction, and simplify your life. Remove all unnecessary material possessions and keep the ones with sentimental value. Try to clear your schedule and only prioritize tasks that are aligned with your values. Refine your goals and reduce them; keep two goals on your list at all times. Only after you have achieved one goal will there be room to add another one.

Expel negative thoughts from your mind and only allow positive ones to remain. Make a plan to reduce your debt so that you can achieve financial independence. Be a woman of few words and try to keep conversations truthful and simple; do not gossip. Keep the food you eat basic and as natural as possible. Cut out your screen time so that you can be more present in your environment, which will encourage mindfulness. Unplug from the world every now and then so that you can attend to the things that are important. Do one thing at a time, and avoid multitasking. Practicing these principles will declutter your life and keep it simple enough to clear your mind as well.

SETTING BOUNDARIES

Black women have to deal with so much in their personal lives and they are expected to do so consistently, be it emotionally, physically, or financially. Black women are not expected to have boundaries, yet they are crucial if somebody wants to maintain emotional self-care. Feeling disgruntled, resentful, and angry could be the result of not knowing how to create and maintain boundaries. Negative feelings will evidently rear their ugly heads if your boundaries are not respected, or you don't have any to begin with.

If you are able to communicate your expectations clearly with another person then you are simultaneously letting them know what you will and will not accept from them and what they should expect from you. There are various types of boundaries, including financial, sexual, physical, intellectual, and emotional boundaries. To set boundaries that will promote self-care for yourself, you have to self-reflect and evaluate why certain boundaries could be important to you. Set your boundaries early in the relationship and be consistent with them.

It is important to keep open lines of communication so that when someone is overstepping your boundaries, you can alert them swiftly. While you set up and enforce your boundaries, it is imperative that you respect and appreciate the boundaries of others. When you constantly cross the boundaries of others, they can resent you for it and avoid you in the future due to your behavior. Respecting another person's boundaries will encourage them to respect yours.

ATTACHMENT

Living a simple life means going through life not attached to anything. In Buddhism, desire is a negative trait, as well as clinging. According to this religion, what brings true joy is knowing that happiness does not stem from holding onto these possessions tightly, but from letting them go. Unhealthy attachment is the idea that if something happens then it will lead to your happiness. The truth is that it is likely you will be momentarily satisfied, but will begin to desire something different shortly afterward. When you attach yourself emotionally and expect your environment, including the people in it, to act a certain way, you will always be disgruntled.

Do not attach to material things because this will create dependency in those things. You should place all your efforts on trying to let go of your desire and dependency. It is not easy to get to this kind of mindset, where you are not attached to your desire or any material possessions. This will keep your life simple, peaceful, and happy. The universe is constantly changing, and therefore, it doesn't make sense to desire, as you are trying to create a fixed idea of something. Suffering is created when you are clashing with the forces of the universe, which will manifest as negative emotions. Cherish the happy moments and understand the difficult ones will not last forever. Nothing is permanent, do not get attached.

LETTING GO LEADS TO PEACE

It takes practice in order to do away with the habit of attachment. When you are successfully able to detach, you will achieve inner peace. There are some practices that you can do at home in order to learn to let go and reduce your suffering.

1. Your mind will constantly attach itself to previous regrets or future worries, yet when you meditate you force your mind to remain firmly planted in the present. What this means is that your mind will shed any attachments to be in the moment.

2. Be bigger than your narrative and apply compassion to yourself as well as to others. It is only with the warmth of your compassion that will you be able to keep suffering at bay.

3. You may have received some kind of enlightenment but you are still joined to everyone on this earth as you all share in the desire to achieve happiness in your lives, as well as being connected due to everybody undergoing the same suffering.

4. Accept things as they are and appreciate the beauty in them. When you are constantly rejecting the present because you are desiring something else, you are holding on to attachment. Let that go.

5. Eventually, your mind will get to a place that is more expansive and isn't defined by this world's narrow focus. Your mind will no longer just be a place for your attachments and your suffering, but it will be as big as the universe and will have space to observe others' attachments and their suffering as well, as all the beauty that is in our world.

Letting go will give you peace as well as joy. The things that matter are not tangible because material things are temporary. A simple life is the only way that you can combat stress constantly, on a daily basis. It can get tiring to be under chronic stress and frustration, and at some point, your body and mind will need a little tender loving care.

9

HEAL YOUR MIND, HEART, AND SOUL

Healing is an art. It takes time, it takes practice. It takes love.

— MAZA DOHTA

E veryone has set standards for themselves. Whether they are too high or too low remains a topic for another day. We are constantly pushing ourselves to do better and achieve more. The drive that a black woman has is incomparable. You keep giving and keep going until you have nothing left inside you. This is not a bad thing unless it is draining you. This means you have self-drive and motivation.

You may be constantly correcting yourself and having private conversations without yourself about your progress and all the things you could have done better. This inner voice that you use to speak to yourself is either giving constructive criticism or it could be tearing you down. You may have a harsh critic you use for inner dialogue. If your inner voice has statements such as, 'You can do it'; 'Nothing can stop you'; 'You are competent'; or 'You will always succeed no matter what', your inner critic will likely be your stepping stone to success.

If your inner monologue is riddled with statements about all the things that you will do wrong or how you are going to fail at something, then you will struggle to be confident. You may get to a point where your criticisms become self-fulfilling prophecies. You know that your thoughts play a big role in your emotions and behaviors. With this constant negative critique, it will be difficult to conquer your fears and maintain a higher level of self-worth. It can be easy to fall into a pattern where we over-criticize ourselves.

If you recognize that you are one of those people that hold themselves to a harsh and critical standard, you can work on this inner voice that is full of self-doubt and inaccuracies. You can reframe your negative inner critic that has been unhelpful to you in the past. Below you will find a short exercise where you can observe your inner voice and possibly reshape it.

CONQUERING YOUR NEGATIVE INNER CRITIC

- **Become aware of your thoughts:** Sometimes we are not aware of what we sound like when we speak to ourselves. Write down what you think or a statement you have said to yourself. Thinking something isn't conclusive evidence that it is true and your thoughts may be disproportionate or biased.

- **Stop dwelling:** Repeating your mistakes over and over in your mind is like reliving an embarrassing moment. Do not ruminate over something questionable you did. Accept that it happened and distract yourself with other activities that make you feel good

- **Advise like a friend:** When we speak to our loved ones, we use a tone of compassion and empathy. We won't come from a place of judgment and will rarely be harsh toward our friends. Instead, we often reassure them that this one-time mistake is not what will define them. This is the same tool we should use toward ourselves; be compassionate, empathetic, and kind toward yourself.

- **Check out the evidence:** If your thoughts are leaning toward the negative side, what may be beneficial to you is to look at all the evidence that supports this negative assertion as well as the evidence that refutes it. Write down each on a piece of paper and eventually you will be able to assess the situation from a less emotional viewpoint.

- **Find accurate statements to replace critical thought:** If your thoughts are exaggerated toward the negative then try to think of a more accurate statement. For example, if you are constantly thinking that you may never find love, change that thinking to you have not found love yet.
- **Envision mishap:** If you entertain your negative thoughts, think about if they came true, would it be a complete catastrophe or would you recover from it? Thinking of the worst-case scenario might make you realize that you can get through it if it should happen, and it will increase your confidence and keep the worry at bay.
- **Accept your flaws and work to improve them:** Striving for self-improvement is not the same as putting yourself down. Always remind yourself that you can do better while accepting your flaws and the things that you struggle with.

You can get in your own way if you are bringing yourself down and not being your own source of motivation. Keep your inner critic at bay in order to cripple your negative thoughts. You are doing the best you can so you should coach yourself in a way that will make you more productive.

FOCUS ON YOUR STRENGTHS AND WHAT YOU DO RIGHT

The best kind of motivation comes from everything within yourself and identifying what you are good at. Capitalizing on the strengths that you already have and improving upon them can give you a new level of satisfaction. Identifying your strengths will make you feel valuable and unique; this will heighten your sense of fulfillment and spur you to go on. Ask those around you that you trust and respect what your strengths could be. Looking into your personality type can also help you get a better understanding of yourself and where your strengths lie.

After recognizing what your strengths are, it is important to refrain from comparing yourself with those around you or in similar positions. Instead of comparing, you could align yourself with people you envy or who will challenge your growth. The people around you also have their strengths; try to use any opportunity you have to learn from their strengths. Having a variety of viewpoints and perspectives will strengthen personal progress.

List Your Strengths

Over the next few days, write down all of the strengths that you think you have in one column. In another column write down all the strengths that your loved ones have listed. Which list has more strengths? When you compare the two columns, which strengths come up a lot?

Keep a Success Journal

Often, we focus on the things that we could have done right or that we always do wrong. This keeps us in a negative mindset. I challenge you to keep a success journal where you record your daily successes. Constantly recording all the things you did right will reshape what you think about yourself; when you look back and recognize the things you have succeeded at, you will look at yourself differently.

SPEND TIME WITH THE MOTIVATORS

You are the company you keep. If you surround yourself with people who have no ambition and who ridicule you for wanting better for your life, you will think you don't deserve to have better. When you are surrounded by people that do not motivate you, people that tear you down, you will remain in the negative headspace that hinders you from overcoming and being productive. On the contrary, if you spend time with people who act as your personal motivators, you become motivated to do better.

Surround yourself with the people who celebrate you. Spend time with those that build you up and want to see you succeed. You need these kinds of people to give you a confidence boost based on facts, especially on days when your emotions and thoughts keep you down. Being with those who build you up will also reshape how you view yourself. If they are constantly seeing the good in you, that is how you will see yourself. Because you believe them when they tell you all the good things about yourself, you will also believe the good things about yourself when they come from your inner monologue.

PERSPECTIVE—GET SOME

It is easy to lose perspective when your life is bombarded with stress and negative emotions. Putting things into perspective can balance your emotions and allow you to shed anxiety and unnecessary worry. When you feel yourself getting overwhelmed by everything that you have on your plate, reconnecting with your life purpose can give you renewed drive. Get in touch with the things that inspire you so that you are not stuck in all the things that are wrong with your current situation. There is a life beyond what is happening to you right now.

Try to keep an open mind and use the power of *yes*. Take a cue from improvisation comedy: When you say yes to everything that is happening and that could happen, you are allowing yourself to be flexible, creative, and visionary. You are not perfect and life is not black and white. Experiences happen more on a gradient and there's more *sometimes* than there is *never* or *always*. Mistakes are essential to your success as they are what you use as lessons to be better.

To gain a better perspective, you can try to put yourself in someone's shoes to see the situation from another viewpoint. When you place your situation in the bigger picture by zooming out on it, check which details actually make a difference in the larger scheme of things and focus on those things. Some things are worthy of obsession in order to get right and some things really don't matter.

START SMALL THEN GO BIG

Imagine if you started with studying for your master's degree or your PhD before you obtained your bachelor's degree. It would be a huge undertaking where you set yourself up for failure. Putting the cart before the horse is not going to get you anywhere. Small effort in the short term will lead to big success in the long term. Therefore, do not start with the big tasks in order to succeed, but rather invest in the small actions first before trying something big.

In the example above, it makes sense to first pursue a bachelor's degree in your desired field, graduate, and then pursue a postgraduate degree. During your bachelor's degree, you will learn how to write academically, how to research topics, and all the little things that will propel you toward success after graduation. When you take on small challenges and succeed at them, this will give you the confidence needed to go for bigger challenges.

PUT YOURSELF FIRST

Putting yourself first before everything is something that is counterintuitive for black women. This is because we have been conditioned to believe that being selfish about our self-care is not a desirable trait. You deserve nothing but the best and, whether it is desirable or not, it is essential to your emotional well-being to prioritize yourself and your self-care above all else. Putting yourself first will allow you to be the best version of yourself a lot of the time. Invest in self-development so that you can keep growing.

Prioritizing yourself means letting go of the expectations that others have put on you. You will not always be able to live up to them, but it is worse if you keep disappointing yourself. Do not think of putting yourself first as selfish, but rather as essential to feeling motivated and energized. Dismantle limiting beliefs that you have come to rely on; you are not a failure, you are not lazy, you aren't anything that prohibits your self-development. Learn how to explore yourself and get curious about your passions and what makes you tick.

Emotional self-care requires a lot of introspection and reevaluation. A lot of the work is internal and will be between you, a pen, and a piece of paper. But emotional self-care is not only concerned with how you feel and the thoughts that are in your mind. Taking care of your body is an essential aspect of emotional self-care. You do not exist only as a concept or soul, you are a physical being as well, and that is a part of you that you cannot ignore. To complete your emotional self-care journey, you must also take care of your physical being.

GOOD HEALTH LEADS TO A GOOD MOOD

Don't wait around for other people to be happy for you. Any happiness you get you've got to make yourself.

— ALICE WALKER

SELF-LOVE

The best way to show yourself love is to show yourself some self-care. Black women are expected to care for their families, their friends, their extended families, and even strangers; no one tells them how to care for themselves. From a young age, you were groomed to be strong and not to complain about anything. But if you keep pouring into others and not into yourself, you won't have any love left for yourself.

Love begins within you. Showing yourself love is how you learn to love in the first place. If you do not know how to love yourself, it is unlikely you will be able to love others. With all the expectation that are placed on black women, you cannot afford to lack self-love. You will still be put in situations where you have to give a lot to other people; if you are not giving yourself love and replenishing regularly, then you will be left feeling frustrated and burnt out.

PHYSICAL SELF-CARE

Your body plays a big role in your emotional stability and resilience. Everything that has to do with your body and your mind is intertwined; you will not be able to achieve emotional well-being if you are not taking care of your physical health. Things like your mental health and mood are tied to what you do to take care of your physical body. Not eating a balanced diet can lead to issues such as obesity, diabetes, and other chronic illnesses. This will affect your self-esteem and self-image.

There are various aspects of your physical health that can lead to you gaining stability in your emotions. It is not just about one perfect thing, but about creating a balance that will give you a holistic approach to your health. Taking the time to put these building blocks in place will ensure that your physical health is in the best condition. Doing the following things will get you closer to being in a better condition physically.

Quality Sleep

Quality sleep is essential to your overall health. It allows your body to rest and repair itself. Interruptions in sleep affect you negatively and can be a contributing cause to certain mental health issues. You may not always be able to control the factors that disrupt your good night's sleep, but you can incorporate certain habits into your life that will improve your quality of sleep.

- Make a sleep schedule that you abide by every single night that does not exceed eight hours. Make sure that you will go to sleep and wake up at the same time every day so that your body learns a consistent sleep-wake cycle; use the same times even on the weekend. If you're finding it harder to sleep, try to do something that will relax you and prepare you for bed, such as listening to calming music or taking a warm bath.
- Try not to go to sleep shortly after eating a large meal or when you are hungry. Allow a few hours between your supper and bedtime. Substances such as caffeine, alcohol, and nicotine might take some time to wear off and will disrupt your sleep.

- Naps during the day can cause interruptions in your sleep at night. A nap shouldn't last more than an hour and should be done in the early afternoon instead of later in the day.
- Physical activity should be a part of your daily routine but should only take place in the morning instead of close to bedtime. Being outside will also assist the quality of your sleep.
- Do not wait until bedtime to think of solutions to your worries, as this will keep you up longer than what you expect. Jot your worries down for the next day and commit to solving them when you wake up.

If you become sleep-deprived, you may accumulate a sleep deficit. As the days pass you may think that you are fine, but at some point, your body will want you to correct this deficit and you'll likely crash. Signs of sleep deprivation include drowsiness, mood changes, trouble focusing, forgetfulness, and falling asleep immediately as you lay down. When you are getting enough sleep, you will feel happy, healthy, productive, and never feel sleepy during the day.

The consequences of not getting enough sleep include having a slower reaction time, being irritable, and feeling a lack of motivation. There are some people who do not get enough sleep who also experience problems with their memory, or they may feel depressed and have a low sex drive. Bad decision-making, or even having problems with making decisions, can come about as consequences of lack of sleep. If you have ever seen people who rarely sleep, they will have dark circles under their eyes and wrinkled skin. Unfortunately, lack of sleep also increases the risk of non-communicable diseases such as high blood pressure, heart disease, diabetes, and obesity.

Sleep deprivation is very dangerous and should not be something that continues to happen in your life. If the quality of your sleep is not improved by the suggested activities above, then perhaps it is time to seek medical intervention. There may be an underlying medical condition that is the cause of your sleep deprivation.

Building a Healthy Plate

A big part of being healthy is eating a healthy diet. Not only does the diet need to be healthy, but it also needs to be balanced. By balanced it means that it should include the right amount of every type of food. During each meal, half of your plate should be fruits and vegetables, a quarter of your plate should be whole grains, and the other quarter of your plate should be protein. Whole grains include food such as barley, whole wheat, quinoa, oats, and brown rice. Protein is found in nuts, poultry, beans, and fish; try to limit red meat, sausages, and bacon.

Healthy plant oils should be used instead of hydrogenated oils; this includes oils such as olive, soy, corn, and canola. Prioritize drinking water over any other beverage; milk and dairy products should be limited to up to two servings daily.

Avoid sugary and fizzy drinks. Another aspect that can improve your physical health is the health of your gut. Ensuring that you eat a diet that has diverse bacteria will improve your overall health. The research surrounding gut health is ongoing, but it seems that it affects numerous areas of our physical well-being.

Exercise for Good Health

Good health is not just about sleep and eating but it also includes exercise. There are so many ways that you can exercise in order to boost your mood and how you feel about yourself. When you are working out, your body is releasing endorphins in your brain. Endorphins assist in stress relief and affect your mood in a positive way. You only need to exercise for no less than 30 minutes, every other day, exerting medium effort. The more endorphins that you have in your brain, the more likely your mental health will be in a good place.

Exercise impacts your mental health in a variety of ways and has been shown to treat depression, anxiety, and stress. Regular exercise has been shown to reduce the symptoms associated with ADHD. Exercising while being mindful can shake your nervous system and snap you out of the paralyzing stress response which is associated with trauma or PTSD. You will sleep better, have a clearer mind, and become more energized when you exercise regularly. In order to boost your mood, try the following exercises:

1. **Lifting weights:** Strength training will improve your mood due to the endorphins that are released in your brain. This is an exercise that can be done anywhere, even at home. If you don't overexert yourself, you can engage in weightlifting five times a week.

2. **Aerobics:** Cardio activities assist in the release of serotonin, which is a mood-boosting hormone. Aerobic exercises include swimming, jogging, or dancing; walking or running on a treadmill is also counted as aerobics. Do not push yourself too hard and always take a break when your body needs a rest.

3. **Tai chi:** This is a martial arts form that originates from Chinese traditions. Tai chi coordinates your movement with your breathing by synchronizing them in a way that promotes the release of endorphins in your brain. When you practice tai chi over a long period of time it may improve your mental health, how you deal with stress, and your overall self-esteem. You will need an instructor who is certified when you first begin practicing tai chi.

4. **Yoga:** This low impact exercise will boost your mood, as it requires meditation and mindful breathing. The more deep breaths you inhale, the more oxygen is delivered to your brain, which will calm your nerves and regulate your emotions. When you are a beginner, it is better to use online videos or an instructor in order to guide you on how to breathe correctly during yoga.

Being Outside

Natural surroundings can serve as a healer when your energy is off balance and you are struggling emotionally. Spending time outside has been shown to reduce your stress levels and anxiety while also lessening symptoms that may be associated with depression. Being outside will also reduce the release of cortisol and lower your heart rate, blood pressure, and muscle tension. You need to feel the sun shining on your face and the fresh air that comes with a crisp breeze. Vitamin D that comes from the sun is crucial to your health.

Spending some time in nature can include hiking, a picnic in your local park, a walk on the beach, camping outside, or walking your dog in a natural environment. My personal favorite is cloud-gazing while lying on the ground and watching them emerge and change as the wind moves them along. Being in nature is a great experience, whether you are on your own or with your family.

YOUR SELF-CARE ROUTINE

In order to make sure that you are adequately caring for yourself, try to keep a record for one week and notice where you might be falling short. On your tracking sheet you should have rows that are labeled from Monday to Sunday. There should be a column for sleep, exercise, nutrition, time outside, and social interaction. The goal of this exercise is to be mindful of the choices you make. Under the sleep column, record the amount of time you slept. Under the exercise column, record what exercise you did and for how long.

With regard to nutrition, you can record whether you had breakfast, lunch, or dinner by using the first letter of those words. If those meals were nutritious, you can circle those letters. Under the outside column, you should record the things that you did outside and for how long you did them. Lastly, under the social interaction column you should write what social activity you were a part of and who you did it with, as well as for how long. When you see what choices you make on paper, it will become glaringly obvious where you're falling short. You will then know what you can do in which area in order to boost your health and stabilize your moods and emotions.

CONCLUSION

My message for everyone's the same: that if we can learn to identify, express, and harness our feelings, even the most challenging ones, we can use those emotions to help us create positive, satisfying lives.

— MARC BRACKET

Emotions are not an easy thing to face. Sometimes they reveal things about ourselves that we are not yet ready to face. Working through difficult emotions is not something that anyone looks forward to. We duck, dive, and maneuver in order to avoid dealing with how we feel about certain things. Some people get so good at avoiding their emotions that they reach the point where they can't deal with them without help. The more you avoid your feelings, the more they will disrupt your life.

The human experience includes various feelings, and it would be unhealthy to go through life avoiding these feelings and opting to feel nothing. You are encouraged to lead a healthy life where you don't need to run from your emotions. Experiencing the spectrum of emotions that come with life is essential to the human experience; emotions are healthy and natural. You create more damage and destruction to your psyche when you shut down. Shutting your emotions out is not healthy and is something you should not attempt to do.

Whether they are good or bad, your emotions are like a compass that guide you in the right direction. Your emotions act as a helpful tool to guide you away from situations that do not bring you peace and toward happiness and success. When you equip yourself with the right skills, you are able to use your emotions in a way that will guide you toward a happier life. Fortunately, this book has given you the foundation you need to stop avoiding your feelings and shown you how to use them to become a well-rounded, content adult.

As a black woman you have to deal with a lot of microaggressions, as well as sexist oppression. There is so much on your plate; therefore, you should not ignore your emotional self-care. Our emotions are power and they should be used as a tool that will reveal more about ourselves. Get to know your feelings and why you feel how you feel. After being able to identify your emotions, you can process and release them. Once those emotions are released, you can then turn to reshaping your thoughts and core beliefs in order to eliminate the harmful ones.

Mindfulness allows us to remain in the present and not to be overwhelmed by negative thoughts and emotions. You gain improved focus and awareness of self when you do things mindfully. You can't run from bad feelings, and it is important not to try to conquer everything in one day. Taking things day by day makes life more manageable. In the end you truly have to focus on healing your mind, heart, and soul by focusing on your strengths and gaining some perspective.

When you succeed at little things, you are motivated and have more vigor to go for bigger things. Emotional self-care is not only about feelings and thoughts, but it also encompasses maintaining good health so that you can remain in a good mood. Make sure that keeping your emotional self-care on the right track is a priority every day so that you can maintain a high level of emotional stability and regulation. Coping is the key to getting through life and succeeding at it.

Embracing your emotions will heal you from past trauma. Living a life of running from what you feel will only create more problems instead of solving the ones you already have.

Any pain that you have within you will be released and this will create a space for light and a rebirth. Recognize emotional self-care for what it is: an opportunity to begin again.

To review this book, you can:

Step 1:

Scan the QR-code below with the camera on your phone to go directly to the review page.

Or type in the Shorturl link below the QR-code in your internet browser.

Step 2:

Give the book a star rating and write your review.

shorturl.at/BFHVX

We appreciate your support!

REFERENCES

Alvarado Parkway Institute. (2016, September 14). Emotional regulation: What is it and why is it important? Alvarado Parkway Institute. https://apibhs.com/2016/09/14/emotional-regulation-what-is-it-and-why-is-it-important#

American Psychological Association. (2014). Depression. APA Dictionary of Psychology. https://dictionary.apa.org/depression

APA Dictionary of Psychology. (n.d.). Anger. APA Dictionary of Psychology. https://dictionary.apa.org/anger

Babauta, L. (2016, March 2). The zen habits guide to letting go of attachments. Zen Habits. https://zenhabits.net/attachments/

Barclays Bank. (n.d.). What are your strengths? 5 ways to find out. Barclays Life Skills. https://barclayslifeskills.com/i-want-to-choose-my-next-step/school/5-ways-to-find-out-what-you-re-good-at/

Barre Body. (2016, August 28). How (and why) to prioritise self care. Barre Body. https://barrebody.com.au/blog/prioritise-self-care/

Becker, J. (n.d.). The 10 most important things to simplify in your life. Becoming Minimalist. https://www.becomingminimalist.com/the-10-most-important-things-to-simplify-in-your-life/

Bee Well Living. (n.d.). 5 mindfulness exercises you can try today. Bee Well Living. https://beewell-living.com/5-mindfulness-exercises-you-can-try-today

Beesley, K. (2018, August 29). Why it's important to get to the root of your emotions. Psychology Today. https://www.psychologytoday.com/us/blog/psychoanalysis-unplugged/201808/why-it-s-important-get-the-root-your-emotions

Bell, J. (n.d.). 4 helpful workouts to boost your mood. Support in Mind Scotland. https://www.supportinmindscotland.org.uk/news/4-helpful-workouts-to-boost-your-mood

Bernstein, R. (2016, July 26). The mind and mental health: How stress affects the brain. Touro University WorldWide. https://www.tuw.edu/health/how-stress-affects-the-brain/

Center for Clinical Interventions. (n.d.). Improving self-esteem improving self-esteem developing balanced core beliefs improving self-esteem module 8: Developing balanced core beliefs improving self-esteem. Center for Clinical Interventions. https://www.cci.health.wa.gov.au/-/media/CCI/Consumer-Modules/Improving-Self-Esteem/Improving-Self-Esteem---08---Developing-Balanced-Core-Beliefs.pdf

Cherry, K. (2020, September 1). What is meditation? Verywell Mind. https://www.verywellmind.com/what-is-meditation-2795927

Cherry, K. (2021, April 5). The 6 types of basic emotions and their effect on human behavior. Verywell Mind. https://www.verywellmind.com/an-overview-of-the-types-of-emotions-4163976#

Chia, S. (2021, February 3). 15 ways to improve your focus and concentration skills. Better Up. https://www.betterup.com/blog/15-ways-to-improve-your-focus-and-concentration-skills

Christensen, D. (2010). Primary and secondary emotions. https://cornercanyoncounseling.com/wp-content/uploads/2015/05/Primary-and-Secondary-Emotions.pdf

Dahl, M. (2016, November 11). 3 ways to channel your raging emotions into action. The Cut. https://www.thecut.com/2016/11/3-ways-to-channel-your-raging-emotions-into-action.html

Demetre, D. C. (2020, September 26). The 7 habits of highly serene people. Science Beta. https://sciencebeta.com/7-habits-serenity/

Dix, M., & Klein, E. (2022, June 24). Improve gut health: Recognize the signs of an unhealthy gut. Healthline. https://www.healthline.com/health/gut-health#improving-gut-health

Dowd-Higgins, C. (n.d.). Be more mindful: 7 tips to improve your awareness. Ellevate Network. https://www.ellevatenetwork.com/articles/6170-be-more-mindful-7-tips-to-improve-your-awareness

Hackspirit. (2017, April 9). Zen buddhism explains why attachments lead to suffering (and what you can do about it). Hack Spirit. https://hackspirit.com/zen-buddhism-attachments-lead-suffering-can/

Harris, S. (2021, February 10). Reframing our thoughts to have positive feelings. AllHealth Network. https://www.allhealthnetwork.org/colorado-spirit/reframing-our-thoughts-to-have-positive-feelings/

Harvard University. (2019). Healthy eating plate. The Nutrition Source. https://www.hsph.harvard.edu/nutritionsource/healthy-eating-plate/

Hicks, B. (2007, March 2). How to make and use a feelings chart. The Kid Counselor®. https://www.thekidcounselor.com/how-to-make-and-use-a-feelings-chart/

Holland, K. (2018, September 24). 20 ways to fight depression. Healthline. https://www.healthline.com/health/depression/how-to-fight-depression#meditation

Idealist. (2021, June 22). 6 strategies for gaining perspective. Idealist. https://www.idealist.org/en/careers/6-strategies-for-gaining-perspective

Itani, O. (2021, April 21). You are what you think: How your thoughts create your reality. Omar Itani. https://www.omaritani.com/blog/what-you-think#

Jennifer. (2021, May 11). 11 life-changing journaling tips for beginners. Simply + Fiercely. https://www.simplyfiercely.com/journaling-tips/

Kapur, A. (2020, September 16). These 8 tips from a top psychologist will help you stay calm in stressful situations. Healthshots. https://www.healthshots.com/mind/mental-health/these-8-tips-from-a-top-psychologist-will-help-you-stay-calm-in-stressful-situations/

Kids Health. (2018). 5 ways to know your feelings better (for teens). Kids Health. https://kidshealth.org/en/teens/emotional-awareness.html

Kos, B. (2020, April 9). The "not-to-do list": A personalized list of tasks and habits you should never do | Spica. Www.spica.com. https://www.spica.com/blog/not-to-do-list#

Lamothe, C. (2019, December 18). How to release anger: 11 tips for letting go. Healthline. https://www.healthline.com/health/how-to-release-anger#ask-for-help

Livingston, M. (2021, June 7). The healing power of holistic medicine and tools used to optimize health. Parsley Health. https://www.parsleyhealth.com/blog/holistic-approach-tools/

Marteka. (2019, July 15). 12 ways to recognise negative thoughts. Benevolent Health. https://benevolenthealth.co.uk/12-ways-to-recognise-negative-thoughts/

Mayo Clinic. (2018, February 3). Depression (major depressive disorder). Mayo Clinic. https://www.mayoclinic.org/diseases-conditions/depression/symptoms-causes/syc-20356007

Mayo Clinic Staff. (2020, April 17). 6 steps to better sleep. Mayo Clinic. https://www.mayoclinic.org/healthy-lifestyle/adult-health/in-depth/

sleep/art-20048379

McCarty, K. (2020, August 19). 5 benefits of mindfulness for black, indigenous, and women of color. Mindful. https://www.mindful.org/5-benefits-of-mindfulness-for-black-indigenous-women-of-color/

Memorial Sloan Kettering Cancer Center. (2019). Acupressure for stress and anxiety. Memorial Sloan Kettering Cancer Center. https://www.mskcc.org/cancer-care/patient-education/acupressure-stress-and-anxiety

Merriam-Webster. (2019). Definition of serene. Merriam-Webster. https://www.merriam-webster.com/dictionary/serene

Miller Law Group. (2021, April 6). Understand the root cause of triggering emotions. Miller Law Group. https://miller-law.com/how-to-drill-down-to-understand-the-root-cause-of-triggering-emotions/

Miller, L. (2020, February 13). How to identify your emotional needs in the moment and verbalize them. Holistic Psychotherapy Boulder. https://www.holisticpsychotherapyboulder.com/my-blog-therapist-in-boulder/how-to-identify-your-emotional-needs-in-the-moment-and-verbalize-them

Mindful. (2020, February 26). How to meditate. Mindful. https://www.mindful.org/how-to-meditate/#how

Mindful Staff. (2020, July 8). What is mindfulness? Mindful. https://www.mindful.org/what-is-mindfulness/

Mindfulness homework: seeing thoughts as thoughts. (n.d.). https://www.bowdoin.edu/counseling/pdf/seeing-thoughts-as-thoughts.pdf

Morin, A. (2014, November 6). Taming your inner critic: 7 steps to silencing the negativity. Forbes. https://www.forbes.com/sites/amymorin/2014/11/06/taming-your-inner-critic-7-steps-to-silencing-the-negativity/?sh=71fdabfa7feb

Parry, G. (2014, December 5). You are not your thoughts and feelings, and they don't have to bring you down. Tiny Buddha. https://tinybuddha.com/blog/living-right-now-you-are-not-your-thoughts-and-feelings/

Patek, A. (n.d.). Using A feelings chart to teach emotions. Generation Mindful. https://genmindful.com/blogs/mindful-moments/using-a-feelings-chart-to-teach-emotions

Paterson, R. (2022, June 15). Think less and grow rich. Think Less and Grow Rich. https://www.thinklessandgrowrich.com/you-are-not-your-thoughts/

Pattemore, C. (2021, June 3). 10 ways to build and preserve better boundaries. Psych Central. https://psychcentral.com/lib/10-way-to-build-and-preserve-better-boundaries

Pejerrey, S. (n.d.). 25 awesome feelings chart ideas | feelings, feelings chart, feelings and emotions. Pinterest. Retrieved June 20, 2022, from https://www.pinterest.com/spejer/feelings-chart/

Primary and secondary emotions. (n.d.). The Emotion Compass. https://emotioncompass.org/information/primary-secondary-emotions/

Princing, M. (2021, September 3). What is toxic positivity? Right as Rain by UW Medicine. https://rightasrain.uwmedicine.org/mind/well-being/toxic-positivity

Product Plan. (n.d.). The 4 ds of time management. Product Plan. https://www.productplan.com/glossary/4-ds-of-time-management/

Psychological & Counseling Services. (2020, April 2). My self-care routine: Daily tracking sheet. University of New Hampshire. https://www.unh.edu/pacs/my-self-care-routine-daily-tracking-sheet

Psychology Tools. (n.d.). Fight or flight response. Psychology Tools. https://www.psychologytools.com/resource/fight-or-flight-response/#

Rachel Reiff Ellis. (2017, June 15). Tips for living with anxiety. WebMD. https://www.webmd.com/anxiety-panic/anxiety-tips

Ragland, L. (2020, November 24). Stress management. WebMD. https://www.webmd.com/balance/stress-management/stress-management

Raypole, C. (2019, November 21). How to deal with toxic people: 17 tips. Healthline. https://www.healthline.com/health/how-to-deal-with-toxic-people#be-unavailable

Raypole, C. (2020a, July 30). Hey you! Quit hiding your feelings. Healthline. https://www.healthline.com/health/mental-health/hiding-feelings#finding-help

Raypole, C. (2020b, November 23). Get over guilt with these steps. Healthline. https://www.healthline.com/health/mental-health/how-to-stop-feeling-guilty#guilt-as-a-tool

Raypole, C. (2021, January 29). Drawing for anxiety: Benefits, easy exercises, & more. Healthline. https://www.healthline.com/health/mental-health/anxiety-drawing#benefits

Ridsdel, J. (2021, April 1). 10 common negative thinking patterns and 5 steps for change. Family Centre. https://www.familycentre.org/news/post/10-common-negative-thinking-patterns-and-5-steps-for-change

Robertson, K. (2021, May 26). Psychedelic therapy: Uses, how it's done, risks, and more. Healthline. https://www.healthline.com/health/mental-health/psychedelic-therapy

Robinson, L., Segal, J., & Smith, M. (2021, August). The mental health benefits of exercise. Help Guide. https://www.helpguide.org/articles/healthy-living/the-mental-health-benefits-of-exercise.htm

Roxburgh, L., & Willard, J. (2016, September 15). How to release tension & stress in the body. Goop. https://goop.com/wellness/fitness/where-stress-gets-stuck-in-the-body-and-how-to-release-it/

Scott, E. (2020, July 13). How to make mindfulness your way of life. Verywell Mind. https://www.verywellmind.com/mindfulness-exercises-for-every day-life-3145187#

Subterranea, H. (2020, May 20). 9 steps to healing chronic anger. Medium. https://medium.com/invisible-illness/9-steps-to-healing-chronic-anger-3e911da5cc84

Suicide Call Back Service. (n.d.). Nature as a healer. Suicide Call Back Service. https://www.suicidecallbackservice.org.au/mental-health/nature-as-a-healer/ .

Team Tony. (2021, July 30). 5 ways to start prioritizing yourself today. Tony Robbins. https://www.tonyrobbins.com/mind-meaning/how-to-priori tize-yourself/

Tension, Stress and Trauma Release : TRE®. (n.d.). Tension & trauma releasing exercises. Tension, Stress and Trauma Release : TRE®. https://traumaprevention.com/

The Master Philosopher. (2017, November 3). How to transform uncomfort-able emotions & find the root of your problems. Medium. https://medium.com/@MasterPhilosopher/how-to-transform-uncomfortable-emotions-find-the-root-of-your-problems-d28e9f31f376

Therapist Aid. (2014). My Fears (Worksheet). Therapist Aid. https://www.therapistaid.com/therapy-worksheet/my-fears

Therapist Aid. (2018). Coping skills: Anger (worksheet). Therapist Aid. https://www.therapistaid.com/therapy-worksheet/coping-skills-anger/anger/none

Therapist Aid. (2020). What are core beliefs? Therapist Aid. https://www.ther
apistaid.com/worksheets/core-beliefs-info-sheet.pdf

Thomas, J. (n.d.). Primary and secondary emotions: What's the difference?
Rumie. https://learn.rumie.org/jR/bytes/primary-and-secondary-
emotions-what-s-the-difference

University of Nevada, Reno. (n.d.). Releasing stress through the power of
music. University of Nevada, Reno. https://www.unr.edu/counseling/
virtual-relaxation-room/releasing-stress-through-the-power-of-music#

UPMC HealthBeat. (2021, May 13). What are cognitive distortions? (With 10
examples). UPMC HealthBeat. https://share.upmc.com/2021/05/cogni
tive-distortions/

Villines, Z. (2017, October 19). Cryotherapy: Safety, what to expect, and benefits. Medical News Today. https:// www.medicalnewstoday.com/articles/
319740#benefits

WebMD. (n.d.-a). How much sleep do I need? WebMD. https://www.webmd.
com/sleep-disorders/sleep-requirements#:

WebMD. (n.d.-b). Stress symptoms: Effects of stress on the body. WebMD.
https://www.webmd.com/balance/stress-management/stress-symptoms-
effects_of-stress-on-the-body#

Wim Hof Method. (n.d.). Cryotherapy. Wim Hof Method. https://www.
wimhofmethod.com/cryotherapy#:

Winfrey, O. (2021, July 25). Oprah says this one act can change the way you
move through the world. Oprah Daily. https://www.oprahdaily.com/life/
a37117486/oprah-forgiveness/

Wolff, C. (2016, March 21). 8 healthy ways to release negative emotion, so you
can feel better the right way. Bustle. https://www.bustle.com/articles/
151298-8-healthy-ways-to-release-negative-emotion-so-you-can-feel-
better-the-right-way

Womens Media. (2021, June 1). How to listen to your feelings as messengers.
Forbes. https://www.forbes.com/sites/womensmedia/2021/06/01/how-
to-listen-to-your-feelings-as-messengers/?sh=36a858103154

Yale. (n.d.). Focus on your strengths, focus on success. It's Your Yale. https://your.
yale.edu/work-yale/learn-and-grow/focus-your-strengths-focus-success

Zimmerman, P. (2019, June 11). How emotions are made. Noldus. https://
www.noldus.com/blog/how-emotions-are-made#